DR. SEBI

TREATMENT & CURE FOR CANCER MADE SIMPLE

Natural Healing Approach to Detoxify, Claense and Boost Alkaline Level to Stop And Degenerate Cancer Cells

JACOB MORRIZ

Copyright© 2024 JACOB MORRIZ

All rights reserved. No part or portion of this book or publication may be reproduced, stored, or transferred in any form by electronic, mechanical, recording, or other retrieval system without permission in writing from the publisher.

CONTENTS

CHAPTER 1 5
    Introduction to Dr Sebi's Philosophy 5

CHAPTER 2 9
    Understanding Cancer 9

CHAPTER 3 16
    The Importance of Nutrition in Healing The Effects of Diet on Cancer 16

CHAPTER 4 23
    Alkalinity and Health 23

CHAPTER 5 29
    PlantBased Nutrition 29

CHAPTER 6 36
    Herbal remedies 36

CHAPTER 7 43
    Detoxification Protocols 43

CHAPTER 8 49
    Fasting for Cancer Recovery 49

CHAPTER 9 56
    Holistic Lifestyle Changes 56

CHAPTER 10 63
    Emotional and Mental Wellbeing 63

CHAPTER 11 70

Recipes and Menu Plans 70

CHAPTER 13 76
Combating Certain Types of Cancer 76

CHAPTER 14 81
Supplemental Practices 81

CHAPTER 15 88
Future Directions in Natural Healing 88

CHAPTER 1

Introduction to Dr Sebi's Philosophy

The Life and Legacy of Dr. Sebi

Dr. Sebi, born Alfredo Darrington Bowman in Honduras in 1933, is a wellknown herbalist, healer, and champion for natural medicine. His introduction to the area of holistic medicine came out of personal necessity. Dr. Sebi struggled with a variety of health concerns, including asthma, diabetes, and impotence, and traditional treatment provided no help. This personal health problem prompted him to seek alternative therapeutic methods.

Dr. Sebi traveled extensively in his search for wellbeing, studying plant therapeutic capabilities. He was especially influenced by indigenous healing traditions from Africa, Central America, and the Caribbean. During these encounters, he gained a thorough awareness of the relationship between nutrition, natural herbs, and total health.

Dr. Sebi's study was based on the assumption that many ailments are caused by the accumulation of mucus and acidity in the body. He contended that keeping the body's pH alkaline was essential for disease prevention and treatment. To back up this view, he developed the "Dr. Sebi Diet," which emphasizes plantbased, alkaline meals.

Dr. Sebi was a lifelong supporter of nature's therapeutic power. He founded the USHA Healing Village in Honduras, a resort where people could detoxify and heal with his direction. Despite criticism and legal challenges, including a wellknown court battle in New York in which he successfully defended his claim of treating AIDS, Dr. Sebi's popularity soared. He became an inspiration to many people looking for alternative health solutions, establishing a legacy that continues to influence the holistic health movement today.

FUNDAMENTAL PRINCIPLES of NATURAL HEALING

Dr. Sebi's concept is based on five essential ideas that serve as the foundation for his natural healing technique. These principles not only guide his dietary recommendations, but also serve as a broader framework for understanding health and disease.

1. Alkaline Environment: Dr. Sebi believed that the body required an alkaline environment to function properly. He claimed that diseases thrive in acidic conditions, which are frequently the result of eating processed meals, sweets, and animal products. Eating alkaline meals, particularly plantbased, can lower acidity in the body and create unfavorable conditions for disease growth.

2. Cellular Nutrition: According to Dr. Sebi, true health starts at the cellular level. He emphasized the necessity of eating natural, whole foods that contain the nutrients required for cellular regeneration and repair. He contended that synthetic supplements and processed foods do not have the same bioavailability or therapeutic potential as natural, plantbased diets.

3. Detoxification: Detoxification is an essential component of Dr. Sebi's treatment routine. He felt that poisons collected from a bad diet, environmental pollution, and stress slowed the body's natural healing processes. Regular detoxification by fasting, herbal medicines, and a healthy diet is required to eliminate these toxins and restore health.

4. Herbal Medicine: Dr. Sebi frequently employed herbal medicine to supplement his dietary advice. He identified several herbs that he thought may cleanse and invigorate the body. These herbs were chosen because of their natural detoxifying properties, capacity to support organ function, and general vitality.

5. Holistic Approach: Dr. Sebi's concept goes beyond physical health and includes mental and emotional wellbeing. He felt that stress, unpleasant emotions, and mental clutter might all lead to physical problems. Thus, his method included techniques aimed at gaining mental clarity and emotional equilibrium, as well as an understanding of the interdependence of mind, body, and spirit.

HOW DR. SEBI'S APPROACH DIFFERS FROM CONVENTIONAL MEDICINE

Dr. Sebi's approach to health and healing differs significantly from mainstream medicine in several respects. Understanding these distinctions is critical to appreciate the unique value and perspective his approaches provide.

1. Holistic vs. Symptomatic Treatment: Conventional medicine frequently focuses on treating symptoms rather than addressing the underlying causes of illness. Pharmaceutical medications and invasive procedures are commonly used as treatments to ease discomfort. In contrast, Dr. Sebi's holistic approach seeks to address the root causes of sickness, such as poor nutrition and toxin buildup. His approach, which focuses on nutrition and natural therapies, aims to restore overall balance and health rather than simply treating symptoms.

2. Natural medicines vs. drugs: Dr. Sebi aggressively pushed for the use of natural, plantbased medicines rather than synthetic drugs. He contended that pharmaceutical medications frequently cause negative effects and even exacerbate existing health issues. Natural therapies, on the other hand, work in tandem with the body's organic processes, facilitating recovery while avoiding side effects.

3. DietCentric Healing: While mainstream medicine frequently downplays the importance of diet in disease prevention and treatment, Dr. Sebi made it the focal point of his healing philosophy. He felt that eating an alkaline, plantbased diet may prevent and even cure many chronic ailments. This emphasis on diet as medicine demonstrates a key distinction between his approach and current medical methods.

4. Preventive Focus: Dr. Sebi's methods are primarily preventive, with the goal of maintaining health and avoiding disease through lifestyle choices. Conventional medicine frequently focuses on treating ailments once they have formed. Dr. Sebi's method aims to prevent disease by encouraging a nutritious diet, regular cleansing, and mental wellbeing.

5. Patient Empowerment: Dr. Sebi underlined the necessity of people having an active role in their own health. His teachings encourage people to make informed decisions about their diet and lifestyle, instilling a sense of personal responsibility and control over their health. This contrasts with the more passive role that patients frequently take in traditional medical systems, where they rely primarily on doctors' prescriptions and treatments.

6. MindBody Connection: Dr. Sebi recognized the strong relationship between mental, emotional, and physical wellness. He incorporated methods that promote mental and emotional wellbeing, understanding that a healthy mind leads to a healthy body. Conventional medicine is gradually recognizing this link, although it has traditionally concentrated on physical symptoms and treatments.

CHAPTER 2

Understanding Cancer

What is cancer?

Cancer is a broad term that refers to a group of diseases marked by the uncontrolled proliferation and spread of aberrant cells. If the spread is not controlled, it can lead to death. Cancer can develop practically anyplace in the human body, which contains trillions of cells. Human cells normally develop and divide to produce new cells as needed by the body. When cells get old or damaged, they die and are replaced by new cells.

Cancer develops when this orderly process breaks down. Cells become increasingly aberrant, with old or damaged cells surviving when they should have died and new cells forming when they are not needed. These excess cells can continue to divide indefinitely, becoming tumors. Tumors can be benign or malignant (cancerous). Malignant tumors can infect surrounding tissues and spread to other parts of the body via the blood and lymphatic systems, a process known as metastasis.

Cancer is more than one disease. There are over 100 forms of cancer, and they are frequently called after the organs or tissues where they develop. For example, lung cancer begins in the cells of the lung, but brain cancer begins in the cells of the brain. Cancers can also be classified by the type of cell that produced them, such as an epithelial cell or a squamous cell.

THE MAJOR CATEGORIES OF CANCER ARE:

Carcinomas are the most frequent type of cancer. They are made up of epithelial cells, which cover both the interior and exterior surfaces of the body. Adenocarcinoma, basal cell carcinoma, and squamous cell carcinoma are the names given to cancers that start in different types of epithelial cells.
Sarcomas are cancers that develop in bones and soft tissues such as muscle, fat, blood vessels, lymph vessels, and fibrous tissue.

Leukemias are cancers that begin in the bone marrow's bloodforming tissue. These cancers do not produce solid tumors. Instead, aberrant white blood cells accumulate in the circulation and bone marrow, displacing normal blood cells.

Lymphomas: Cancers that originate in the lymphatic system (the tissues and organs that manufacture, store, and transport white blood cells that fight infections).

Multiple Myeloma is a cancer that develops in plasma cells, which are immunological cells.

Melanomas: Cancers that begin in cells that develop into melanocytes, which are responsible for the color of skin.

Understanding cancer biology entails investigating how alterations in cells cause the disease. Cancer research is ongoing, with the goal of identifying the complex causes and mechanisms that lead to more effective prevention, diagnosis, and therapy.

COMMON CAUSES AND RISK FACTORS

Cancer can be caused by a number of circumstances, many of which occur together. While the actual etiology of cancer is unknown, many risk factors have been linked to an increased risk of developing the disease. These risk factors are classified into four categories: lifestyle, environmental, genetic, and biological.

1. Lifestyle Factors:

Tobacco Use: Smoking is the major cause of lung cancer and has been related to a variety of other cancers, including the mouth, throat, bladder, pancreas, and stomach. Tobacco use is a major risk factor for cancer, accounting for roughly onethird of all cancer deaths.

Diet and Physical Activity: A diet high in processed foods and red meats, but low in fruits and vegetables, can raise the risk of numerous cancers, including colorectal cancer. Physical inactivity and obesity have been related to an increased risk of breast, endometrial, and colon cancer.

Alcohol Consumption: Drinking alcohol increases the chance of developing malignancies of the mouth, throat, esophagus, liver, breast, and colon. The danger rises with the amount of alcohol ingested.

2. Environmental Factors:

Carcinogen Exposure: Cancercausing substances are known as carcinogens. Environmental exposure to certain chemicals and poisons can raise the risk of developing cancer. Examples include asbestos, benzene, formaldehyde, and certain insecticides.

Radiation: Cancer can be caused by both ionizing radiation (such as radon gas, xrays, and gamma rays) and nonionizing radiation (such as UV rays from the sun or tanning beds). Ionizing radiation can cause DNA mutations that lead to cancer, whereas UV radiation is the primary cause of skin malignancies, such as melanoma.

3. Genetic factors:

Inherited Mutations: Some people inherit genetic mutations from their parents, which dramatically raises their risk of developing certain cancers. For example, mutations in the BRCA1 and BRCA2 genes have been associated with an increased risk of breast and ovarian cancer.

Family History: A family history of specific cancers may indicate a hereditary risk. It is crucial to remember that, while a family history can increase the risk of developing cancer, it does not ensure it.

4. Biological factors:

Age: As people age, their risk of having cancer increases. This is due in part to the accumulation of cell damage over time, and the body's ability to heal this damage decreases with age.

Viruses and Infections: Some infections are associated with an increased risk of cancer. Human papillomavirus (HPV) has been related to cervical and other cancers, hepatitis B and C to liver cancer, and Helicobacter pylori infection to stomach cancer.

Hormones: Hormonal changes, particularly in women, can affect cancer risk. Longterm exposure to estrogen and progesterone, whether from early menstruation, late menopause, or hormone replacement therapy, raises the risk of breast cancer.

Understanding these risk factors is critical for cancer prevention and identification at an early stage. Lifestyle changes such as stopping smoking, eating a balanced diet, maintaining a healthy weight, and protecting oneself from damaging UV radiation can dramatically lower cancer risk. Awareness of family history and genetic predispositions can also result in proactive surveillance and early intervention.

Conventional vs. Holistic Treatments

Conventional medical techniques to cancer treatment have long dominated, with surgery, chemotherapy, radiation therapy, and targeted therapies being the most common. However, holistic treatments, which include a larger range of activities, are gaining favor as complementary and alternative solutions. Understanding the distinctions, benefits, and limitations of these approaches can assist patients in making informed judgments regarding their treatment options.

Conventional Treatments:

1. Surgery is frequently the first line of treatment for many solid tumors. The goal is to remove the tumor and, if required, some healthy tissue around it in order to eliminate all cancerous cells. Surgery may be curative, particularly if the cancer is identified early and has not spread.

2. Chemotherapy: Chemotherapy is the use of chemicals to kill or inhibit the division of cancer cells. These medications can be given orally or intravenously, and they move through the bloodstream to cancer cells throughout the body. Chemotherapy is commonly used for tumors that have spread (metastasized), and it can be combined with other treatments such as surgery or radiation.

3. Radiation Therapy: Highenergy particles or waves are used to kill or harm cancer cells. It can be given either externally (external beam radiation) or internally (brachytherapy). Radiation therapy focuses on specific locations, making it beneficial for confined tumors.

4. Targeted Therapy: This modern strategy uses medications or other substances to directly target cancer cells while causing minimum damage to healthy cells. These medicines target specific molecules involved in cancer growth and progression. Examples include monoclonal antibodies and tyrosine kinase inhibitors.

5. Immunotherapy: Immunotherapy tries to strengthen the body's natural defenses against cancer. It employs chemicals produced by the body or in a laboratory to boost or restore immune system function. Examples include checkpoint inhibitors and CAR Tcell therapy.

HOLISTIC TREATMENTS:

Holistic treatments focus on the patient's total wellbeing, including physical, emotional, and spiritual health. These treatments are frequently used in conjunction with traditional therapy to help the body's natural healing processes and improve overall quality of life.

1. Diet and Nutrition: Holistic approaches frequently emphasize the value of a balanced diet in cancer treatment and prevention. Diets high in fruits, vegetables, whole grains, and lean proteins can provide vital nutrients for the immune system and overall health. Specific dietary regimens, such as Dr. Sebi's alkaline diet, seek to produce an environment in the body that is less conducive to cancer development.

2. Herbal Medicine: Many holistic practitioners employ herbal treatments to help cancer patients. Herbs such as turmeric, green tea, and garlic have been investigated for their anticancer qualities. These natural compounds can help to strengthen the immune system, reduce inflammation, and protect cells from injury.

3. Detoxification: Detoxification procedures seek to eliminate toxins from the body, which can benefit overall health and potentially improve the efficacy of traditional cancer treatments. Dietary detoxes, herbal cleanses, saunas, and colon hydrotherapy are all options.

4. MindBody Techniques: Stress management and emotional wellbeing are critical components of integrative cancer care. Meditation, yoga, acupuncture, and massage treatment are all effective ways to relieve stress, increase mood, and boost the body's inherent healing capacities.

5. Exercise and Physical Activity: Regular physical activity is recommended as part of a comprehensive cancer treatment plan. Exercise can improve physical function, reduce weariness, and boost mental health. It can also aid with weight management and lower the chance of cancer recurrence.

COMPARISON AND INTEGRATION:

While traditional treatments primarily target cancer cells and tumors, holistic treatments try to strengthen the body's natural defenses and improve overall health. Both techniques have advantages and disadvantages, and many healthcare providers prefer an integrative strategy that blends the best of both worlds.

Effectiveness
& Side Effects: While conventional therapies can be extremely effective in decreasing or eliminating cancer, they are frequently associated with substantial side effects such as nausea, exhaustion, and hair loss. While holistic treatments are generally gentler on the body, they may not be sufficient to treat severe malignancies on their own, but they can help alleviate adverse effects and enhance quality of life.

Personalized Care: Holistic treatments frequently stress personalized care, taking into account the patient's general lifestyle, interests, and values. Conventional treatments generally adhere to conventional protocols, but personalized medicine approaches, such as genetic analysis, are increasingly being used to adapt therapy.

Supportive Care: Integrative oncology, a combination of traditional and unconventional treatments, is becoming more popular. This method seeks to provide holistic care that covers both cancer therapy and the patient's general health. A patient receiving chemotherapy, for example, may receive nutritional counseling, acupuncture to reduce side effects, and stressreduction strategies such as meditation.

Patient Empowerment: Holistic treatments frequently encourage patients to take an active role in their health care, promoting lifestyle modifications and selfcare habits with longterm benefits. Traditional treatments, while successful, can occasionally leave patients feeling inert or overwhelmed by the medical system.

CHAPTER 3

The Importance of Nutrition in Healing The Effects of Diet on Cancer

The link between nutrition and cancer is extensive, and knowing it is critical for both prevention and therapy. Numerous studies have revealed that nutrition influences cancer risk, development, and recurrence. Diet affects cancer through a variety of pathways, including inflammation, oxidative stress, hormone control, and immunological function.

1. Inflammation: Chronic inflammation has been linked to a variety of cancers. Diets high in processed foods, red and processed meats, refined carbohydrates, and bad fats can all cause inflammation in the body. Antiinflammatory diets, on the other hand, include fruits, vegetables, whole grains, and healthy fats such as nuts and olive oil. Reducing inflammation through food can reduce the chance of cancer formation and improve the body's ability to combat existing cancer.

2. Oxidative Stress: Oxidative stress is caused by an imbalance between free radicals and antioxidants in the body. Free radicals can damage DNA, proteins, and cell membranes, resulting in cancer. Plantbased meals include numerous antioxidants, which neutralize free radicals and minimize oxidative stress. Antioxidantrich diets, such as vitamins C and E, selenium, and phytochemicals, help protect cells and lower the risk of cancer.

3. Hormone Regulation: Certain diets can alter hormone levels in the body, thereby increasing the risk of cancer. Highfat diets and obesity, for example, have been related to elevated levels of estrogen and insulin, hormones that can encourage the formation of malignancies such as breast and prostate cancer. Plantbased diets rich in fiber and low in fat can help regulate hormone levels and lower cancer risk.

4. Immune Function: The immune system is crucial in recognizing and eliminating cancer cells. A balanced diet promotes immune function by supplying necessary foods such as vitamins, minerals, and phytochemicals. For example, vitamin D, zinc, and selenium are required for a strong immunological response. Diets low in these nutrients can impair the immune system and raise cancer risk.

5. Microbiome Health: New study emphasizes the role of the gut microbiome in overall health, including cancer risk. A diversified and balanced microbiome promotes immune function, decreases inflammation, and aids in the detoxification of possible carcinogens. Diets strong in fiber, fermented foods, and prebiotics support a healthy microbiome, whereas diets high in processed foods and low in fiber upset microbial balance and raise cancer risk.

Epidemiological studies corroborate these theories by demonstrating a link between food and cancer incidence. For example, populations that consume a lot of fruits, vegetables, and whole grains had lower cancer rates than those who eat a lot of processed foods and red meat. The Mediterranean diet, which is high in plantbased foods, healthy fats, and lean meats, has been linked to a reduced risk of cancer and other chronic diseases.

DR. SEBI'S NUTRITIONAL PHILOSOPHY

Dr. Sebi's nutritional philosophy is founded on the concept that maintaining an alkaline environment in the body is critical for disease prevention and treatment, including cancer. His approach stresses eating natural, plantbased foods while avoiding processed foods, animal products, and synthetic drugs. Dr. Sebi's theory is heavily anchored in cellular nutrition, detoxification, and a holistic view of health.

1. Alkaline Diet: An alkaline diet is central to Dr. Sebi's theory, which holds that it can help prevent and cure ailments. He said that many diseases, including cancer, thrive in an acidic environment, which is frequently the outcome of eating processed foods, sweets, and animal products. Eating alkaline foods, primarily raw fruits, vegetables, nuts, and seeds, can reduce acidity in the body and create unfavorable conditions for disease progression.

2. Natural and Whole Foods: Dr. Sebi promoted the intake of whole, unprocessed foods. He felt that natural foods are most useful when they remain undisturbed by human intervention. Processed foods, which frequently contain artificial additives, preservatives, and refined sugars, are viewed as harmful to health. Dr. Sebi's diet focuses on foods that are as close to their natural state as possible.

3. Herbal Medicine: In addition to diet, Dr. Sebi included herbal medicine in his nutritional philosophy. He identified several herbs that he thought may cleanse and invigorate the body. These herbs were chosen because of their natural detoxifying properties, capacity to support organ function, and general vitality. Burdock root, sarsaparilla, and bladderwrack are all known for their cleansing and immuneboosting effects.

4. Detoxification: Dr. Sebi's technique relies heavily on detoxification. He felt that poisons collected from a bad diet, environmental pollution, and stress slowed the body's natural healing processes. Regular detoxification by fasting, herbal medicines, and a healthy diet is required to eliminate these toxins and restore health. This method cleanses the body at the cellular level, boosting overall health and illness prevention.

5. Holistic Approach: Dr. Sebi's concept goes beyond physical health and includes mental and emotional wellbeing. He felt that stress, unpleasant emotions, and mental clutter might all lead to physical problems. Thus, his method included techniques aimed at gaining mental clarity and emotional equilibrium, as well as an understanding of the interdependence of mind, body, and spirit. Meditation, deep breathing, and spending time in nature were recommended to improve general wellness.

Dr. Sebi's nutritional philosophy is comprehensive, aiming to address health at its core. His method focuses on food, purification, and holistic activities in order to create an internal environment that promotes the body's inherent ability to heal itself.

CREATING A CANCERFIGHTING DIET

A cancerfighting diet consists of foods and behaviors that enhance the body's ability to prevent and resist cancer. This diet focuses on nutrientdense, plantbased meals that provide important vitamins, minerals, and antioxidants. The following are major components and practical instructions for developing a diet that promotes cancer prevention and treatment.

1. Emphasize PlantBased Foods: A plantbased diet includes plenty of fruits, vegetables, whole grains, legumes, nuts, and seeds. These foods contain critical nutrients, fiber, and phytochemicals that promote general health and lower cancer risk. Specific plantbased foods with strong anticancer qualities include:

　Cruciferous Vegetables: Broccoli, cauliflower, Brussels sprouts, and kale contain substances known to suppress cancer cell development and promote detoxification, such as sulforaphane and indole3carbinol.

　Berries: Blueberries, strawberries, and raspberries include antioxidants such as vitamin C and ellagic acid, which protect cells from damage and inflammation.

　Leafy Greens: Spinach, Swiss chard, and arugula are high in vitamins, minerals, and fiber, which promote immune function and detoxification.

　Nuts and Seeds: Almonds, walnuts, flaxseeds, and chia seeds all include healthy fats, fiber, and phytochemicals that promote heart health and lower inflammation.

2. Incorporate Healthy Fats: Healthy fats are beneficial to general health and can help reduce inflammation. Sources of healthful fats include:

　Omega3 Fatty Acids are found in flaxseeds, chia seeds, walnuts, and fatty seafood such as salmon. Omega3s are antiinflammatory and can help prevent cancer.

　Monounsaturated fats are found in avocados, olive oil, and nuts. These fats promote cardiovascular health and minimize inflammation.

3. Avoid Processed Foods: Processed foods are high in harmful fats, refined sugars, and artificial additives, which can lead to inflammation and cancer risk. Foods to avoid are:

Refined Sugars and Grains: White bread, pastries, sugary drinks, and snacks can raise blood sugar levels and induce inflammation.

Processed Meats: Bacon, sausage, and deli meats have been linked to an increased risk of colorectal cancer due to high levels of preservatives and harmful fats.

Trans Fats: Trans fats, which are found in many fried and packaged foods, can cause inflammation and increase the risk of heart disease and cancer.

4. Hydration and Detoxification: Staying hydrated promotes general health and assists the body in eliminating toxins. Drinking plenty of water, herbal teas, and eating waterrich meals such as fruits and vegetables will help in detoxification. Specific detoxifying foods include:

Lemon and lime: These citrus fruits help to alkalize the body and aid in liver cleansing.

Green Tea: High in antioxidants, green tea promotes detoxification and has been linked to anticancer effects.

5. Herbs and Spices: Adding herbs and spices to your diet can improve flavor and bring additional health advantages. Herbs and spices that can help fight cancer include:

Turmeric: Curcumin, a potent antiinflammatory and antioxidant substance, can prevent cancer cell proliferation.

Garlic: Contains sulfur compounds that aid in detoxifying and have been demonstrated to lower the incidence of some malignancies.

Ginger: Has antiinflammatory characteristics and can help alleviate nausea caused by cancer therapies.

6. Fasting and Intermittent Fasting: Fasting and intermittent fasting can both aid in detoxification and cellular restoration. These practices include times of restricted eating, which can help reduce inflammation, aid in weight management, and boost the body's natural healing processes.

An Example CancerFighting Meal Plan: Breakfast:
Green smoothie made with spinach, kale, blueberries, flaxseeds, and almond milk.

A handful of raw nuts (almonds, walnuts)

Lunch: Quinoa salad with chickpeas, cherry tomatoes, cucumbers, and avocado, topped with olive oil and lemon juice.

Fresh fruit, such as an apple or pear.

Snack: Carrots and celery sticks with hummus.

Herbal tea (green tea, ginger tea)

Dinner: Baked salmon with roasted Brussels sprouts and sweet potatoes.

Mixed berry salad sprinkled with chia seeds

Dessert Options include fresh fruit or a modest dish of dark chocolate (70% cocoa or higher).

Building a cancerfighting diet entails making informed decisions about the foods we consume and how they can benefit our general health and wellbeing. By focusing on nutrientdense, plantbased foods, healthy fats, and avoiding processed foods, we may develop a diet that not only lowers the risk of cancer but also promotes the body's natural healing power.

Practical Tips for Implementing a CancerFighting Diet

Implementing a cancerfighting diet can be both simple and satisfying. Here are some practical strategies for incorporating these nutritional guidelines into your daily life:

1. Plan and Prep Meals: Planning meals ahead of time and preparing ingredients will help you stick to a healthy diet. Batchcooking healthy grains, chopping veggies, and prepping snacks ahead of time can help you save time and avoid the temptation to eat harmful meals.

2. Shop Smart: Make a shopping list for cancerfighting foods and stick to it. Shop the periphery of the grocery store, where fresh produce, nutritious grains, and lean proteins are usually found. Avoid aisles containing processed and packaged goods.

3. Read Labels: Before purchasing packaged goods, carefully read the labels to avoid additional sugars, bad fats, and artificial ingredients. Look for items with few ingredients that are organic or nonGMO.

4. Cook at Home: Cooking at home gives you more control over the ingredients and serving amounts. Experiment with fresh recipes and cooking methods to make healthy eating fun and sustainable.

5. Stay Hydrated: Carry a reusable water bottle and aim to drink at least eight glasses of water each day. Waterrich fruits and vegetables, as well as herbal teas, can help keep you hydrated.

6. Listen to Your Body: Notice how different foods make you feel. Everybody is unique, so what works for one person may not work for another. Adjust your diet to meet your own health needs and preferences.

7. Seek Help: Adopting a new diet might be tough. Seek assistance from friends, family, or a healthcare professional who knows your objectives and can offer advice and encouragement.

8. Mindful Eating: Enjoy each bite, eat carefully, and pay attention to hunger and fullness signs. This can aid digestion and reduce overeating.

CHAPTER 4

Alkalinity and Health

The Science of Alkaline Diets

The alkaline diet is based on the theory that particular meals can change the body's pH equilibrium, hence influencing general health. The pH scale, which ranges from 0 to 14, determines how acidic or alkaline a thing is. pH 7 is considered neutral. The human body has a tightly controlled pH balance, with blood normally having a slightly alkaline pH of around 7.4.

1. Understanding pH Balance: The kidneys, lungs, and blood buffering systems all help the body maintain pH balance. The kidneys maintain pH by excreting excess acids or bases, whereas the lungs do so by regulating the quantity of acidic carbon dioxide in the blood. Buffering systems, such as bicarbonate, aid to neutralize acids and bases in bodily fluids.

2. Diet and pH Levels: What we eat can affect the pH of our urine and, to a lesser extent, our blood. Foods are classified as acidforming or alkalineforming according to how they affect the body's pH after digestion and metabolism. Meat, dairy, cereals, and processed meals are acidforming, whereas the majority of fruits, vegetables, nuts, and seeds are alkaline.

3. Metabolic Processes: When the body digests food, it produces a "ash" residue that might be acidic or alkaline. When proteins and grains are digested, they produce sulfuric and phosphoric acid, which results in an acidic ash. In contrast, fruits and vegetables metabolize to create bicarbonate, resulting in an alkaline ash. This residue affects the body's overall acidbase balance.

4. Health Implications: Proponents of the alkaline diet think that eating more alkalineforming foods can improve health by lowering the body's acid load, which is thought to help prevent diseases like cancer. They argue that an acidic environment in the body can cause chronic ailments, whereas an alkaline environment promotes optimal cellular activity and cleansing.

5. Scientific Evidence: Scientific evidence for the alkaline diet is inconsistent. According to several studies, a diet rich in alkalineforming fruits and vegetables is linked to better health outcomes, such as a lower risk of chronic diseases and better bone health. However, these advantages may be due more to the nutrient density and antioxidant characteristics of these foods than to their effects on pH. There is limited direct evidence that adjusting the body's pH through diet can significantly improve overall health or disease risk.

HOW ALKALINITY AFFECTS CANCER CELLS

The link between alkalinity and cancer cells is a major focus of the alkaline diet research. While the scientific community continues to research this link, various theories and preliminary studies indicate that maintaining an alkaline environment in the body may influence cancer cell activity and overall cancer risk.

1. Cancer Cell Environment: Cancer cells frequently flourish in acidic conditions. Tumors typically establish an acidic microenvironment by altered metabolism, such as enhanced glycolysis, which produces lactic acid even in the presence of oxygen (the Warburg effect). This acidity allows cancer cells to penetrate adjacent tissues, avoid immune detection, and withstand apoptosis.

2. pH and Cancer Growth: Some research suggests that alkalizing the environment around cancer cells can slow their growth and spread. Alkaline environments can alter cancer cell metabolism, diminish their invasiveness, and make them more susceptible to apoptosis. However, these effects are primarily found in vitro (in laboratory conditions) and may not fully translate to the complicated milieu of the human body.

3. Alkaline Diet as Supportive Therapy: While an alkaline diet alone is unlikely to cure cancer, it may help conventional cancer treatments by making the environment less suitable for cancer cells. For example, some integrative oncology techniques propose that an alkaline diet can improve the efficacy of chemotherapy and radiation by making cancer cells more susceptible to these therapies.

4. Acidosis and Overall Health: Chronic lowgrade metabolic acidosis, which is frequently caused by a high acidforming diet, can lead to a variety of health problems such as inflammation, bone demineralization, and decreased muscle mass. These diseases can indirectly influence cancer risk and progression by reducing the body's defenses and general resistance.

5. Limitations and Considerations: It is crucial to remember that while eating a balanced diet high in alkalineforming foods can benefit overall health, it is not a substitute for traditional cancer treatments. The human body possesses robust pHregulating mechanisms, and the diet's influence on blood pH is minimal in comparison to these physiological processes. As a result, an alkaline diet should be seen as a supplementary technique rather than a single treatment.

STEPS TO ACHIEVE AND MAINTAIN ALKALINITY

Achieving and maintaining alkalinity entails following dietary and lifestyle habits that support a balanced pH in the body. Here are some practical strategies to develop and maintain an alkaline environment:

1. Increase your intake of alkalineforming foods: Eat a variety of fruits, vegetables, nuts, seeds, and legumes. Some of the most alkalineforming foods are:

Leafy greens include spinach, kale, and Swiss chard.

Cruciferous vegetables include broccoli, cauliflower, and Brussels sprouts.

Citrus fruits: lemons, limes, oranges (while acidic in nature, they have an alkalizing impact on the body).

Root veggies include carrots, beets, and sweet potatoes.

Nuts and seeds: almonds, chia seeds, and flaxseeds

2. Limit AcidForming items: Reduce your consumption of items that contribute to acidity, such as

Animal proteins include red meat, chicken, and fish.

Dairy goods include milk, cheese, and yogurt.

Processed foods include packaged snacks, processed sweets, and fast food.

Grains: wheat, rice, and oats (moderation is crucial rather than total elimination)

3. Stay Hydrated: Proper hydration promotes kidney function and pH equilibrium. Drink plenty of water all day, aiming for at least eight glasses. Adding a touch of lemon or lime can boost alkalinity.

4. Incorporate Alkaline Beverages: Herbal teas, green tea, and alkaline water can help to maintain alkalinity. Avoid sugary drinks, sodas, and excessive coffee, which can all contribute to acidity.

5. Monitor pH Levels: Use pH test strips to keep track of your body's pH levels. Test your pee or saliva first thing in the morning for the most reliable results. Aim for a slightly alkaline pH (7.0–7.4).

6. Balanced Meals: Make sure that each meal contains a healthy balance of alkalineforming foods. For example, combine protein sources with a variety of vegetables and healthy fats. This equilibrium can help to counteract the acidic effects of proteins and grains.

7. Reduce Stress: Chronic stress can cause acidity in the body. Meditation, deep breathing, yoga, and regular physical activity can all help you reduce stress. Getting enough sleep is also important for keeping a good pH balance.

8. Detoxification: Toxins that cause acid in the body can be eliminated with regular detoxification. Incorporate techniques such as intermittent fasting, drinking detoxifying herbal teas, and eating foods with detoxifying characteristics, such as dandelion greens and beets.

9. Mindful Eating: Eat slowly and chew properly to help digestion and nutrition absorption. Avoid overeating, as it might cause stomach problems and acidity.

10. Supplements: Consider alkaline mineral supplements (e.g., magnesium, potassium, calcium) and green superfood powders. However, it is best to contact a healthcare provider before beginning any new supplement program.

EXAMPLE ALKALINE DIET PLAN:

Breakfast:

Green smoothie made with spinach, kale, avocado, banana, chia seeds, and almond milk.

A handful of raw nuts (almonds, walnuts)

Lunch:

Quinoa salad made with mixed greens, cherry tomatoes, cucumbers, bell peppers, avocado, and lemontahini dressing

Fresh fruits, like a bowl of berries

Snack:

Carrot and celery sticks with hummus

Herbal tea (chamomile or peppermint

Dinner:

Baked salmon served alongside roasted Brussels sprouts and sweet potatoes.

Mixed green salad with olive oil and lemon dressing.

Dessert:

Fresh fruit or a modest portion of dark chocolate (70% cocoa or more)

LIFESTYLE PRACTICES THAT SUPPORT ALKALINITY:

1. Regular Exercise: Regular physical activity promotes general health and reduces stress. Walking, running, swimming, and yoga can all contribute to a healthy pH balance.

2. Adequate Sleep: Make sure you receive 79 hours of good sleep every night. Sleep is essential for recovering and maintaining metabolic equilibrium, which includes pH regulation.

3. MindBody Practices: Use mindbody techniques like meditation, deep breathing exercises, and mindfulness to reduce stress and improve mental health.

4. Avoid Toxins: Reduce your exposure to environmental toxins like cigarette smoke, pollution, and household chemicals, which can all contribute to acidity.

5. healthy Social ties: Keep healthy relationships and social ties, as emotional health has a big impact on general wellbeing and can influence physiological processes.

CHAPTER 5

PlantBased Nutrition

The Power of PlantBased Foods

Plantbased nutrition is at the heart of many modern dietary recommendations due to its multiple health benefits, including the ability to prevent and treat chronic diseases such as cancer. This dietary approach focuses on complete, unprocessed plant foods such fruits, vegetables, grains, nuts, seeds, and legumes, while limiting or eliminating animal products.

1. Nutrient Density: Plantbased foods are high in vital nutrients such as vitamins, minerals, fiber, and phytonutrients. These minerals are essential for overall health and illness prevention. Fruits and vegetables, for example, have significant levels of antioxidants, which protect cells from free radical damage and may reduce the risk of cancer.

2. AntiInflammatory Properties: Chronic inflammation is recognized as a risk factor for a variety of disorders, including cancer. Plantbased diets frequently contain antiinflammatory effects. For example, berries, leafy greens, and almonds contain antiinflammatory chemicals. Omega3 fatty acids present in flaxseeds and chia seeds are also effective antiinflammatory agents.

3. Gut Health: Fiberrich plantbased diets promote a healthy gut microbiome, which is critical for overall health. A diverse and healthy gut microbiome can boost immunity, reduce inflammation, and improve nutrient absorption. Fermented plant foods like sauerkraut, kimchi, and tempeh provide helpful probiotics that improve intestinal health.

4. Detoxification: Many plantbased foods help the body's natural detoxification process. Cruciferous plants, such as broccoli and Brussels sprouts, have chemicals that improve liver function and detoxification pathways. Waterrich fruits and vegetables, such as cucumbers and watermelons, aid in the elimination of toxins from the body.

5. Weight Management: Plantbased diets are frequently lower in calories and higher in fiber than diets high in animal products. This combination can aid in weight management, which is significant because obesity is a risk factor for many types of cancer. Plantbased diets also include fewer saturated fats, which have been linked to an increased risk of cancer.

6. Phytochemicals are bioactive substances found in plants that provide several health advantages. These include flavonoids, carotenoids, and polyphenols, which are antioxidants, antiinflammatory, and anticancer. Lycopene in tomatoes, for example, has been demonstrated to lower the incidence of prostate cancer, whilst sulforaphane in broccoli has been discovered to suppress cancer cell proliferation.

7. Alkalizing Effect: Many plantbased foods have an alkaline pH, which can help keep the body in balance. An alkaline environment in the body is thought to promote health and maybe lower the risk of diseases like cancer. Alkalizing foods include leafy greens, fruits, and nuts.

Essential Nutrients for Cancer Prevention

A wellplanned plantbased diet includes all of the necessary nutrients required for cancer prevention. Here are the essential nutrients and their plantbased sources:

1. Antioxidants:
Vitamin C is found in citrus fruits, strawberries, bell peppers, and broccoli. Vitamin C protects cells against oxidative damage and boosts immunological function.
Vitamin E is found in nuts, seeds, and green leafy vegetables. Vitamin E contains antioxidants that protect cell membranes from harm.
Betacarotene is found in carrots, sweet potatoes, and spinach. Betacarotene is turned to vitamin A in the body, which helps with immunological function and cell growth.
Selenium is found in Brazil nuts, sunflower seeds, and brown rice. Selenium is a potent antioxidant that prevents cell damage.

2. Fiber:

Contains whole grains, legumes, fruits, and veggies. Fiber assists digestion, helps to maintain a healthy weight, and promotes a healthy gut microbiota, all of which are vital in cancer prevention.

3. Phytonutrients:

Flavonoids are found in berries, apples, onions, and tea. Flavonoids contain antiinflammatory and antioxidant effects.

Carotenoids are found in carrots, sweet potatoes, and kale. Carotenoids are antioxidants that may help lower the incidence of some malignancies.

Polyphenols are found in green tea, coffee, red wine, and dark chocolate. Polyphenols have been found to have anticancer effects.

4. Omega 3 Fatty Acids:

Can be found in flaxseeds, chia seeds, walnuts, and hemp seeds. Omega3s lower inflammation and promote heart health, which are essential for overall health and cancer prevention.

5. Vitamins and Minerals:

Vitamin D: Vitamin D is primarily derived by sunlight, but it can also be found in fortified plant milks and supplements. Vitamin D promotes immunological function and bone health.

Magnesium is found in nuts, seeds, leafy greens, and whole grains. Magnesium is involved in more than 300 metabolic events in the body, including DNA repair and immunological function.

Folate is found in leafy greens, legumes, and oranges. Folate plays a critical role in DNA synthesis and repair.

6. Protein:

Required for cellular repair and immunological function. Plantbased protein sources include legumes, lentils, quinoa, nuts, seeds, tofu, and tempeh. A diversified plantbased diet can provide all of the essential amino acids required for good health.

7. Calcium:

Contains fortified plant milks, leafy greens, almonds, and tahini. Calcium is essential for bone health and cell function.

Dr. Sebi's Recommended Food List

Dr. Sebi, a wellknown herbalist and natural healer, advocated a diet high in alkalineforming, plantbased foods to promote health and avoid disease. His recommended diet includes a variety of fruits, vegetables, cereals, nuts, seeds, and herbs. Here's a detailed look at the foods recommended by Dr. Sebi:

1. Fruits:

Apples are high in fiber, antioxidants, and vitamins.

Berries: Fruits including blueberries, strawberries, and raspberries are abundant in antioxidants and vitamins.

Cherries include vitamins, minerals, and antioxidants.

Grapes are high in antioxidants and polyphenols.

Melons: Watermelon and cantaloupe are hydrating and high in vitamins and minerals.

Limes and lemons: Despite their acidic taste, they have an alkalising impact and are abundant in vitamin C.

2. Vegetables:

Leafy Greens: Kale, spinach, and arugula are high in vitamins, minerals, and antioxidants.

Cruciferous Vegetables: This includes broccoli, cauliflower, and Brussels sprouts, which are known for their detoxifying capabilities.

Root Vegetables: Carrots, beets, and sweet potatoes are rich in vitamins and minerals.

Squash: Nutrientdense and versatile squash, such as zucchini and butternut.

3. Grains:

Quinoa: A complete protein with all of the essential amino acids, as well as a high fiber and mineral content.

Amaranth: Rich in protein, fiber, and minerals such as magnesium and iron.

Teff is a glutenfree grain high in protein, fiber, and calcium.

4. Nuts & Seeds:

Almonds are high in healthful fats, protein, and fiber.

Walnuts are high in omega3 fatty acids and antioxidants.

Chia Seeds are high in fiber, omega3s, and other minerals.

Flaxseeds are high in omega3 fatty acids and lignans, which have antioxidant characteristics.

5. Legumes:

Lentils are high in protein, fiber, and vital elements such as iron and folate.

Chickpeas are high in protein, fiber, and vitamins.

6. Herbs and Spices:

Basil: Rich in antioxidants, vitamins, and antiinflammatory qualities.

Oregano is high in antioxidants and has antibacterial effects.

Thyme is known for its antibacterial and antimicrobial properties.

Sage contains antioxidants and antiinflammatory chemicals.

7. Herbal teas:

Dandelion Root: Enhances liver cleansing and overall wellness.

Burdock Root is known for its bloodpurifying qualities.

Sarsaparilla: High in minerals and promotes cleansing.

8. Oils:

Olive Oil: High in monounsaturated fats and antioxidants, which promote heart health.

Coconut Oil: Contains mediumchain triglycerides (MCTs), which boost energy and promote brain function.

Example PlantBased Meal Plan:

Breakfast:

Green smoothie made with kale, spinach, banana, chia seeds, and almond milk.

Fresh berries sprinkled with flaxseeds.

Lunch:

Quinoa salad made with mixed greens, chickpeas, cherry tomatoes, cucumber, avocado, and lemontahini dressing

One serving of fresh fruit, such as an apple or orange.

Snack:

Carrot and celery sticks with hummus

Tea made from dandelion or burdock root

Dinner:

Baked sweet potato served with steamed broccoli and cauliflower.

Mixed green salad with olive oil and lemon dressing.

Dessert:

Fresh fruit or a modest portion of dark chocolate (70% cocoa or more)

HOW TO IMPLEMENT A PLANTBASED DIET:

1. Gradual Transition: Begin introducing more plantbased meals into your diet gradually. This may make the change more doable and sustainable. Begin with "Meatless Mondays" and gradually ramp up the amount of plantbased days.

2. Diverse Foods: Eat a variety of plantbased foods to ensure you get all of your necessary nutrients. Change up your fruits, veggies, grains, and legumes to make meals exciting and healthily balanced.

3. Meal Planning: Plan your meals ahead of time to guarantee a healthy intake of important nutrients. Batchcook grains, legumes, and veggies to have readymade ingredients for quick meals.

4. Flavorful Cooking: Experiment with herbs, spices, and cooking methods to improve the flavor of plantbased dishes. This can make meals more enjoyable and filling.

5. Education and Resources: To guarantee a wellrounded approach, educate yourself on plantbased nutrition and seek out credible resources such as cookbooks, nutrition websites, and guidance from plantbased dietitians.

6. Community Support: Join plantbased communities or seek out a support group. Sharing experiences, recipes, and advice with others can boost motivation and help you overcome obstacles.

7. Mindful Eating: Practice mindful eating by focusing on hunger and fullness cues, savoring each bite, and enjoying the sensory experience of eating.

8. Listen to Your Body: Notice how different foods make you feel. Adjust your diet based on your body's responses and nutritional requirements.

CHAPTER 6

Herbal remedies

Herbal medicine, also known as botanical medicine or phytotherapy, has been used for thousands of years in numerous cultures to prevent and treat sickness. It entails combining plant elements including leaves, roots, flowers, and seeds to make treatments that promote health and wellness. In recent years, there has been a renewed interest in herbal therapy as people seek natural alternatives to traditional therapies, even for serious illnesses such as cancer.

1. Historical Background: Herbal medicine has a long history, stretching back to ancient civilizations in China, Egypt, India, and Greece. Traditional herbal knowledge was frequently passed down through generations, serving as the foundation for early medicinal systems such as Traditional Chinese Medicine (TCM) and Ayurveda. These systems detected the healing characteristics of numerous plants and combined them to generate effective treatments.

2. Scientific Validation: Modern science has begun to validate several traditional herbal applications. Plants include a variety of bioactive chemicals with medicinal potential, including alkaloids, flavonoids, terpenes, and phenolic acids. These chemicals may have antioxidant, antiinflammatory, anticancer, antibacterial, or immunomodulatory properties.

3. Integrative Approach: Herbal medicine can be used in conjunction with conventional treatments to provide an integrative approach to healthcare. Herbs may help cancer patients relieve symptoms, lessen adverse effects from therapies such as chemotherapy and radiation, and enhance their general quality of life. It is critical to utilize herbal treatments under the supervision of a trained healthcare provider to avoid potential problems with conventional pharmaceuticals.

4. Regulation and Safety: The regulations governing herbal medicine vary by nation. In some locations, herbs are categorized as dietary supplements and do not go through the same rigorous testing as

medications. This can result in differences in quality and efficacy. To ensure safety and proper use, herbs should be sourced from trustworthy suppliers and consulted with healthcare professionals.

5. Personalized Medicine: Herbal medicine stresses a patientcentered approach to treatment. When recommending herbs, practitioners typically take into account the individual's particular constitution, health history, and current condition. This comprehensive approach seeks to restore balance and promote the body's natural healing processes.

Top Herbs for Cancer Treatment

Several herbs have been investigated for potential anticancer effects. Here are some of the top herbs recognized for their usefulness in cancer treatment:

1. Turmeric (Curcuma Longa):
Active Compound: Curcumin, turmeric's main active component, has been extensively studied for its anticancer qualities. It has antiinflammatory, antioxidant, and antiproliferative properties.
Mechanism: Curcumin inhibits several cell signaling pathways implicated in cancer development, including apoptosis (programmed cell death), angiogenesis (creation of new blood vessels), and metastasis (the spread of cancer cells). It can also improve the efficacy of chemotherapy while reducing its negative effects.
Usage: Turmeric can be cooked, consumed as a supplement, or applied topically. Combining it with black pepper improves curcumin absorption.

2. Green tea (Camellia sinensis)
Active Compounds: The most prevalent catechin in green tea is epigallocatechin gallate (EGCG), which is renowned for its powerful anticancer activities.
Mechanism: EGCG reduces cancer cell proliferation, causes apoptosis, and inhibits angiogenesis. It also serves as a potent antioxidant, shielding cells from DNA damage.
Usage: Drinking several cups of green tea per day or taking green tea extract supplements can have positive effects.

3. Milk Thistle (Silybum Marianum):

Active Compound: Milk thistle's principal active component is silymarin, a flavonoid group.

Mechanism: Silymarin has antioxidant, antiinflammatory, and anticancer properties. It protects liver cells from poisons and may improve the effectiveness of chemotherapy.

Usage: Milk thistle is usually consumed as a supplement in capsules, pills, or tinctures.

4. Ashwagandha (withania somnifera):

Active Compounds: Ashwagandha's active components are steroidal lactones known as withanolides.

Mechanism: Ashwagandha possesses adaptogenic characteristics, which assist the body cope with stress. It improves immunological function, decreases inflammation, and has the ability to limit cancer cell proliferation.

Usage: Ashwagandha is available in powdered form, pills, and liquid extract.

5. Ginger(Zingiber officinale):

Active components: Gingerol and shogaol are the main active components in ginger.

Mechanism: Ginger has both antiinflammatory and antioxidant effects. It has the ability to limit cancer cell development, induce apoptosis, and improve the efficacy of traditional cancer treatments.

Uses: Ginger can be consumed fresh, dried, or as a supplement. It is also effective at relieving chemotherapyinduced nausea.

6. Garlic (Allium sativum):

Active chemicals: Allicin and other sulfurcontaining chemicals are what give garlic its therapeutic benefits.

Mechanism: Garlic contains strong anticancer, antibacterial, and immuneboosting effects. It suppresses cancer cell proliferation, promotes apoptosis, and may lower the risk of some malignancies.

Usage: Fresh garlic, garlic powder, or supplements may be used. Crushing or cutting garlic and leaving it to sit before cooking boosts allicin production.

7. Astragalus (astragalus membranaceus):

Active Compounds: The main active components of astragalus are saponins, flavonoids, and polysaccharides.

Mechanism: Astragalus strengthens the immune system, improves chemotherapy efficacy, and has anticancer characteristics. It also promotes overall health and resiliency.

Usage: Astragalus is often used in tinctures, capsules, and teas.

8. Echinacea (Echinacea purpurea):

Active Compounds: Alkamides, caffeic acid derivatives, and polysaccharides are the main active ingredients.

Mechanism: Echinacea regulates immunological function, decreases inflammation, and has been investigated for its ability to suppress cancer cell proliferation.

Usage: Echinacea is available in tincture, pill, and tea form.

9. Cat's Claw (Uncaria tomentosa):

Active Compounds: Oxindole alkaloids, glycosides, and tannins are the active ingredients in a cat claw.

Mechanism: Cat claw contains immuneboosting, antiinflammatory, and anticancer effects. It strengthens the body's natural defense mechanisms and may improve the effectiveness of cancer therapies.

Usage: Cat's claw comes in capsule, tincture, and tea form.

10. Reishi Mushroom (Ganoderma Lucidum):

Active Compounds: Triterpenes, polysaccharides, and peptidoglycans are the primary active ingredients.

Mechanism: Reishi mushroom exhibits immunomodulatory, antiinflammatory, and anticancer properties. It improves immunological function, prevents cancer cell proliferation, and promotes general health.

Usage: Reishi can be taken as a tea, tincture, pill, or powder.

Preparing and Applying Herbal Remedies

Herbal treatments must be prepared and used with an understanding of the many methods for extracting and delivering the therapeutic components found in herbs. Here are some popular ways to prepare herbal remedies:

1. Infusions:
 Method: Infusions are created by steeping herbs in hot water, similar to brewing tea. This procedure is appropriate for delicate portions of the plant, such as leaves and flowers.
 Procedure: Add around 12 teaspoons of dry herb or 24 tablespoons of fresh herb to each cup of water. Pour boiling water over the herb, cover, and steep for 10–15 minutes. Strain and drink.
 Examples: Chamomile, peppermint, and nettle are popular infusions.

2. Decoctions:
 Method: Decoctions are made by boiling harder components of the plant, such as roots, bark, and seeds, in water to extract medicinal qualities.
 Procedure: Add around 12 tablespoons of dried herb to 3 glasses of water. Bring the water and herbs to a boil, then reduce the heat and simmer for 2030 minutes. Strain and drink.
 Examples: Ginger root, dandelion root, and licorice root are frequently made as decoctions.

3. Tinctures:
 Method: Tinctures are concentrated liquid extracts obtained by soaking herbs in alcohol or glycerin.
 Process: Fill a glass jar with chopped fresh or dried herbs. Cover the herbs with alcohol (vodka or brandy) or glycerin to ensure they are completely soaked. Seal the jar and keep it in a cold, dark area for 46 weeks, shaking occasionally. Strain the mixture through cheesecloth and place the tincture in a dark glass bottle.
 Dosage: Typically, 12 dropperfuls (approximately 3060 drops) of tincture are taken two to three times a day.
 Examples: Echinacea, astragalus, and milk thistle are common tincture ingredients.

4. Capsules and Tablets:

Method: Capsules and tablets contain powdered herbs or standardized extracts and are a simple way to take herbal treatments.

Procedure: Capsules can be prepared at home with a capsulefilling machine and empty capsules or purchased premade.

Examples: Turmeric, ashwagandha, and garlic are commonly found in capsule form.

5. Topical Applications:

Method: Herbal medicines can be applied directly to the skin in the form of balms, creams, poultices, and compresses to treat certain ailments.

The Procedure:

Salves/Creams: Gently heat herbs in a carrier oil (such as olive oil) until infused. Strain the oil and blend with beeswax to make a salve.

Poultices: Crush fresh herbs or combine dried herbs with a little water to make a paste. Apply directly to the affected region and wrap in a clean cloth.

Compresses: Soak a cloth in a herbal infusion or decoction, then apply it on your skin.

Examples: Topical applications often include calendula, comfrey, and St. John's wort.

6. Herbal oils:

Method: Herbal oils are created by infusing herbs in a carrier oil, which can subsequently be used for massage, salves, or skin moisturizer.

Procedure: Fill a jar with dry herbs and seal with a carrier oil. Seal the jar and store it in a warm, sunny location for 23 weeks, shaking daily. Strain the oil, then keep it in a dark glass bottle.

Examples: Lavender, arnica, and rosemary are popular herbal oils.

7. Herbal Syrup:

Method: Herbal syrups are sweetened, concentrated herbal extracts that are commonly used to treat coughs and colds.

Procedure: Make a decoction with the herbs, filter, and simmer until the liquid has been reduced by half. Add an equal amount of honey or glycerin to the reduced liquid and mix thoroughly. Refrigerate in a glass jar.

Dosage: Typically, 12 teaspoons of syrup are consumed as needed.

Examples: Elderberry and ginger are common ingredients in herbal syrups.

Guidelines for Using Herbal Remedies:

1. Consultation: Always speak with a healthcare practitioner or an experienced herbalist before beginning any new herbal therapy, especially if you have preexisting health concerns or are using other medications.

2. Dosage: Follow the indicated dosages exactly. More is not always better, and certain plants can be harmful in large doses.

3. Quality: For maximum efficacy and safety, choose highquality, organic herbs from reliable sources.

4. Allergies and Sensitivities: Be mindful of any allergies or sensitivities. Start with modest quantities to see how your body reacts to a new plant.

5. Documentation: Keep track of the herbs you use, including their form, dose, and any effects or side effects you notice. This can help you determine what works best for you.

6. Storage: Keep herbal remedies in a cool, dark area to maintain their potency. To keep tinctures and oils from light, store them in dark glass bottles.

CHAPTER 7

Detoxification Protocols

Understanding Detoxification

Detoxification is an essential component of holistic health practices, as stressed by many traditional healing systems, including Dr. Sebi's. The technique entails eliminating toxins from the body in order to improve health and avoid sickness. Understanding the principles and practices of detoxification can assist anyone, particularly cancer patients, in supporting their bodies' natural healing mechanisms.

1. What is detoxification?:

Detoxification is the physiological process by which the body eliminates undesirable chemicals such as environmental contaminants, metabolic waste products, and poisons from food and water. This process predominantly affects the liver, kidneys, intestines, lungs, lymphatic system, and skin.

The liver is the primary detoxification organ, converting poisons into watersoluble molecules that are excreted through urine or bile. The kidneys filter the blood, removing waste products and excess chemicals. The intestines evacuate waste through bowel motions, whereas the lungs release carbon dioxide and other gaseous poisons. Sweating excretes toxins from the epidermis, while the lymphatic system transfers waste materials from tissues to the bloodstream for disposal.

2. The Importance of Detoxification

Regular detoxification is critical for sustaining good health, especially in modern contexts where toxins are pervasive. These toxins can build up in the body, potentially leading to chronic disorders like cancer.

Detoxification strengthens the immune system, improves nutrition absorption, decreases inflammation, and boosts overall organ performance. Detoxification can help cancer patients reduce their toxic load, enhance treatment outcomes, and live a better life.

3. Signs Of Toxic Overload:

Toxic overload symptoms may include chronic fatigue, headaches, digestive troubles, skin problems, hormonal imbalances, cognitive difficulties, and decreased immunity. Recognizing these indications may suggest the need for detoxification.

4. Detoxification and Cancer:

Cancer can be caused by a variety of hereditary, environmental, and lifestyle factors, including toxin exposure. Individuals who assist the body's detoxification pathways may be able to lower their cancer risk and improve their body's ability to fight cancer.

Detoxification can help manage the negative effects of traditional cancer therapies like chemotherapy and radiation, which can introduce new toxins into the body.

DR. SEBI'S DETOX METHODS

Dr. Sebi, a wellknown herbalist and natural healer, pioneered a unique detoxification method based on alkalinity and natural healing principles. His approaches center on detoxifying the body in order to restore balance and encourage healing.

1. The Philosophy of Alkalinity

Dr. Sebi's detox treatments are based on the principle of maintaining an alkaline internal environment. He felt that disease, especially cancer, thrived in acidic environments, and that alkalizing the body may help prevent and reverse illness.

Alkaline foods, which are mostly plantbased, serve to neutralize acidity in the body, reduce inflammation, and promote general health.

2. Fasting:

Fasting is a key component of Dr. Sebi's detox procedures. It entails fasting for a set period of time in order to rest the digestive system and allow the body to focus on detoxification and healing.

Fasting is classified into three types: water fasting (drinking only water), juice fasting (consuming only fresh vegetable and fruit juices), and intermittent fasting.

Fasting can assist to reduce inflammation, improve insulin sensitivity, strengthen the immune system, and improve the body's ability to clear toxins.

3. Herbal teas and tonics:

Dr. Sebi advised the use of various herbal teas and tonics to aid in cleansing. These herbal combinations are intended to cleanse the liver, kidneys, bloodstream, and lymphatic system.

Common plants include burdock root, dandelion root, sarsaparilla, nettle, and chamomile. These plants contain diuretic, antioxidant, antiinflammatory, and immuneboosting effects.

4. Irish moss (Sea Moss)

Sea moss, often called Irish moss, is a form of red algae that Dr. Sebi commonly used in his detox treatments. It contains minerals such as iodine, potassium, calcium, and magnesium, and is said to help with thyroid function, digestion, and immunity.

Sea moss can be ingested as a gel, mixed into smoothies, or taken as a supplement. It cleanses the digestive tract, provides necessary nutrients, and promotes general detoxification.

5. Hydration:

Adequate water is required for efficient detoxification. Water aids in the removal of pollutants through urine, sweat, and bowel movements. Dr. Sebi recommended drinking plenty of pure, alkaline water to aid in the detoxification process.

with addition to water, drinking fresh vegetable and fruit juices can provide hydration and other nutrients to aid with detoxification.

6. Dietary Guidelines:

Dr. Sebi's dietary instructions emphasize eating alkaline, complete, plantbased meals. These meals help the body's natural detoxification processes and supply vital nutrients for recovery.

Leafy greens, fresh fruits and vegetables, nuts, seeds, and whole grains are all important parts of the diet. Avoiding processed meals, sweets, dairy, meat, and artificial additives is critical for lowering the toxic burden on the body.

Practicable Detox Plans for Cancer Patients

Implementing a detox plan can be very advantageous for cancer patients since it supports their therapy and improves their general wellbeing. Here are some useful detox regimens suited to the needs of cancer patients:

1. Initial Preparation:

Before beginning any detox regimen, contact a healthcare physician, particularly for cancer patients undergoing treatment. The detox strategy should be adapted to each person's specific demands and medical problems.

Prepare for detox by progressively limiting your consumption of processed foods, caffeine, alcohol, and sugar. To help with the adjustment, eat more fresh fruits and vegetables and drink more water.

2. 7 Day Detox Plan:

Days 1–2: Fasting

Start with a 12 day juice fast to initiate the detox process. Drink fresh vegetable and fruit juices, herbal teas, and plenty of water.

Recommended juices include green juices (kale, spinach, cucumber, celery), carrotapple juice, and beetrootginger juice.

Herbal teas including dandelion root, burdock root, and chamomile can help the liver and kidneys operate.

Day 3–7: Alkaline Diet:

Switch to an alkaline diet high in fresh fruits, vegetables, whole grains, nuts, and seeds.

Use sea moss gel in smoothies or as a supplement to replenish minerals and aid digestion.

Continue to drink herbal tea and plenty of water.

Example meals include green smoothies for breakfast, salads with leafy greens and avocado for lunch, and steamed veggies with quinoa for dinner.

Snack options include fresh fruit, nuts, and seeds.

3. The 14Day Detox Plan:

Week One: Gradual Transition:

Gradually eliminate processed foods, dairy, meat, and sugar from your diet.

Increase your consumption of fresh fruits and veggies, whole grains, nuts, and seeds.

Start each day with a glass of warm lemon water to promote digestion and detoxification.

Incorporate sea moss gel, herbal teas, and fresh vegetable juice into your everyday regimen.

Week Two: Intensive Detox:

Begin a more thorough detox routine, focusing on raw foods, green juices, and herbal teas.

Practice intermittent fasting by eating all meals within an 8hour period every day.

Dry brush and take Epsom salt baths to promote lymphatic drainage and toxin removal through the skin.

Perform light physical activity, such as yoga or walking, to increase circulation and aid in detoxifying.

4. The 30Day Detox Plan:

Phase 1: Preparation (Days 1–7):

Slowly minimize your intake of processed foods, coffee, alcohol, and sugar.

Increase your intake of fresh fruits, vegetables, and whole grains.

Start each day with a glass of warm lemon water and add sea moss gel and herbal teas.

Phase 2: Deep Cleansing (Days 821):

Eat a strict alkaline diet that focuses on raw and gently cooked plantbased meals.

Incorporate green smoothies, salads, vegetable soups, and steamed veggies into your everyday diet.

Continue to drink herbal teas and fresh vegetable juices.

Practice intermittent fasting and regular physical activity.

Phase 3: Maintenance (Dates 2230):

Adopt a wellbalanced, plantbased diet that you can stick to over time.

Continue to include fresh fruits, veggies, whole grains, nuts, and seeds.

Maintain a consistent intake of sea moss gel, herbal teas, and fresh vegetable juices.

Practice healthy lifestyle habits like frequent exercise, proper sleep, stress management, and hydration.

ADDED DETOX PRACTICES:

1. Liver Cleansing:

The liver is the primary detoxification organ, and it might benefit from specific cleansing techniques.

Consuming liverfriendly foods like beets, carrots, leafy greens, and citrus fruits will help improve liver function.

Herbal supplements such as milk thistle, dandelion root, and turmeric can help the liver detoxify.

2. Colon Cleansing:

A healthy colon is necessary for proper detoxification. Fiberrich diets like fruits, vegetables, whole grains, and seeds promote regular bowel movements and toxin removal.

Drinking plenty of water and consuming herbal teas like senna and cascara sagrada will help cleanse the colon.

3. Skin detoxification:

The skin is a key detoxification organ, and techniques such as dry brushing, sauna sessions, and Epsom salt baths can help toxin excretion through perspiration.

Using natural skincare products and avoiding synthetic chemicals can help to decrease skin toxicity.

4. Lymphatic System Support:

The lymphatic system carries waste items from tissues into the bloodstream for disposal. Supporting lymphatic drainage is essential for detoxification.

Dry brushing, massage, yoga, and regular physical activity can all improve lymphatic flow and purification.

CHAPTER 8

Fasting for Cancer Recovery

The Science of Fasting

Fasting, or abstaining from meals for certain periods of time, has long been a feature of many cultural and religious traditions. In recent years, scientific study has begun to unearth the enormous health benefits of fasting, notably in terms of cancer recovery.

1. Understanding Fasting:

Fasting activates a number of metabolic and cellular processes that can improve health and promote healing. When the body is deprived of meals, it shifts from using glucose as its primary energy source to using stored fats, resulting in ketones. This metabolic transition can cause a variety of physiological effects, including improved cellular repair and reduced inflammation.

2. Cellular autophagy:

One of the primary benefits of fasting is the activation of autophagy, a cellular mechanism that degrades and recycles damaged cellular components. Autophagy aids in the removal of damaged proteins and organelles, which can accumulate and contribute to disease, including cancer.
Fasting promotes autophagy, which aids in cellular renewal and maintenance, improving the body's ability to combat cancer cells and reducing tumor growth.

3. Immune System Enhancement:

Fasting has been linked to improved immune system function. Shortterm fasting can cause a drop in white blood cell count, followed by the regeneration of new, more efficient immune cells upon refeeding. This rejuvenation process can assist the body in better detecting and eliminating cancer cells.

4. Hormonal and Metabolic Changes

Fasting alters hormone levels, which can aid in cancer recovery. For example, fasting lowers insulin and insulinlike growth factor 1 (IGF1) levels, both of which are linked to cancer progression. Lower levels of these hormones can lessen the likelihood of cancer cell proliferation while also improving treatment outcomes.

Fasting also promotes the synthesis of ketones, which serve as an alternate energy source for healthy cells while potentially starving cancer cells that rely on glucose for growth.

5. Lowered Inflammation and Oxidative Stress:

Chronic inflammation and oxidative stress are major contributors to cancer formation and spread. Fasting can assist to reduce inflammation by decreasing the synthesis of proinflammatory cytokines and increasing the release of antiinflammatory chemicals.

Fasting protects cells from DNA damage and other negative consequences that can lead to cancer by lowering oxidative stress.

Types of Fasting Regimens

Fasting regimens vary in terms of protocols and advantages. Individual health problems, tastes, and goals all influence which style of fasting is appropriate. Here are some popular fasting regimens:

1. Intermittent Fasting:

Intermittent fasting (IF) is the practice of eating and fasting alternately over a 24hour cycle. Intermittent fasting can be accomplished by a variety of strategies, including:

16/8 strategy: This strategy entails fasting for 16 hours and eating inside an 8hour window every day. For example, one could eat between 12 and 8 p.m., then fast from 8 to 12 p.m. the next day.

5:2 Diet: This regimen entails eating regularly five days a week and considerably cutting calorie intake (by 500600 calories) on the other two days.

AlternateDay Fasting: This strategy entails alternating between days of normal eating and days of fasting or taking extremely few calories (for example, 500 calories).

Intermittent fasting is simple to implement into daily life and can bring numerous health benefits, such as improved insulin sensitivity, weight loss, and increased cellular repair.

2. Prolonged fasting:

Prolonged fasting is defined as abstaining from all or most food for a lengthy period of time, which can range from 24 hours to several days. This sort of fasting is more rigorous and should be done with caution and under medical supervision, particularly for cancer patients.

24Hour Fast: This entails fasting for an entire 24hour period once or twice every week. For example, one could fast from supper one day until dinner the following day.

48Hour Fast: Fasting for 48 hours can result in greater cellular and metabolic benefits, but it necessitates more preparation and recovery.

72Hour Fast: This lengthy fast can cause significant metabolic changes, such as increased autophagy and immune cell regeneration. It is critical to stay hydrated and gradually reintroduce meals after a fast.

3. The FastMimicking Diet (FMD):

The fastingmimicking diet is a relatively recent concept that entails following an extremely lowcalorie diet (usually 500800 calories per day) for five consecutive days per month. This diet is intended to simulate the metabolic consequences of fasting while delivering critical nutrients.

FMD can provide the benefits of extended fasting without the inconvenience of total food abstinence. It is especially useful for people who require a more reasonable fasting schedule.

4. Water Fast:

Water fasting is the practice of only ingesting water for a defined period of time, which can range from 24 hours to several days. This form of fasting necessitates careful planning and should be overseen by a healthcare expert, particularly for those with medical issues.

Water fasting can cause rapid weight reduction, increased autophagy, and considerable detoxification. However, it can be difficult and may not be appropriate for everyone.

5. Juice fasting:

Juice fasting is the practice of drinking only fresh vegetable and fruit juices for a specific period of time. This sort of fasting replenishes critical vitamins, minerals, and antioxidants while resting the digestive system.

Juice fasting is easier to maintain than water fasting and provides cleansing advantages. Use fresh, organic fruit and avoid sugary liquids.

BENEFITS AND CAUTIONS OF FASTING

While fasting can have various benefits for cancer recovery, it is important to proceed with caution and be aware of potential hazards. Here are the benefits and precautions to take:

1. The Advantages of Fasting for Cancer Recovery:

Enhanced Cellular Repair and Autophagy: Fasting increases autophagy, which aids in the removal of damaged cells and the regeneration of healthy cells. This process is critical for cancer patients because it can help destroy cancer cells and slow tumor growth.

Improved Immune Function: Fasting can strengthen the immune system by encouraging the growth of new, more efficient immune cells. A stronger immune system is better able to recognize and eliminate cancer cells.

Hormonal Regulation: Fasting lowers levels of insulin and IGF1, hormones linked to cancer growth. Lower levels of these hormones can limit the growth of cancer cells and improve therapy results.

Reduced Inflammation: Fasting reduces the generation of proinflammatory cytokines, hence reducing chronic inflammation, which can contribute to cancer formation and progression.

Weight Management: Fasting can cause weight loss and improved body composition, lowering the chance of cancer recurrence and improving general health.

Enhanced Treatment Efficacy: According to some research, fasting can increase the efficacy of traditional cancer treatments like chemotherapy and radiation by making cancer cells more vulnerable to these therapies while sparing healthy cells.

Mental Clarity and Emotional Wellbeing: Many people say that fasting improves their mental clarity and emotional wellbeing, which can be especially beneficial for cancer patients dealing with the stress and emotional toll of their diagnosis and treatment.

2. Precautions and considerations:

Medical Supervision: Cancer patients should always check with their doctor before beginning any fasting regimen. Medical supervision is required to maintain safety and identify potential issues.

Individual Needs: Fasting regimens should be adjusted to individual requirements, taking into account the kind of cancer, stage of treatment, overall health, and nutritional state. What works for one individual may not be right for another.

Hydration: Staying hydrated is critical during fasting periods. Adequate water intake promotes detoxification and prevents dehydration. Electrolyte balance should also be maintained, particularly after extended fasting.

Nutrient Intake: It is critical to maintain enough nutrient intake, especially during extended fasting periods. To avoid deficits, vitamin and mineral supplements may be required.

Potential Side Effects: Fasting may cause dizziness, exhaustion, headaches, or irritability. These symptoms are usually transient and can be treated with adequate preparation and support.

Contraindication: Fasting may not be appropriate for everyone. Individuals with specific medical issues, such as diabetes, eating disorders, or severe malnutrition, should avoid fasting or do so under close medical supervision.

Gradual Transition: It is critical to ease into and out of fasting periods gradually. Sudden food changes can be stressful for the body and have negative consequences.

Implementing Fasting for Cancer Recovery

1. Preparation:

Consultation: First, visit with a healthcare expert to identify the best fasting program. Discuss any potential dangers and create a specific plan.

Gradual Reduction: Reduce your consumption of processed foods, caffeine, sugar, and alcohol in the days leading up to a fast. To help with the adjustment, eat more fresh fruits and vegetables and drink more water.

Mental Preparation: Mentally prepare for the fasting time by setting specific intents and goals. Mindfulness and meditation can help reduce stress and improve the fasting experience.

2. During the fast:

Hydration: Drink plenty of water during your fasting time. Herbal teas and electrolyte solutions may also be effective.

Rest and Relaxation: Make time for rest and relaxation throughout the fast. Avoid intense physical activity and instead favor mild workouts like yoga or strolling.

Monitoring: Keep an eye out for any indicators of side effects, such as extreme exhaustion, dizziness, or other troubling symptoms. Seek medical advice if necessary.

3. Break the Fast:

Gradual Reintroduction: Slowly break the fast by reintroducing easily digestible foods such fresh fruits, vegetables, and soup. Initially, avoid foods that are heavy, processed, or oily.

Mindful Eating: Pay attention to your hunger and satiety indicators. Chew your food properly and appreciate each bite to aid digestion and nutritional absorption.

NutrientDense meals: Choose nutrientdense, whole meals to aid with recovery and overall health. Include a diverse range of fresh fruits, vegetables, whole grains, nuts, seeds, and lean proteins.

Case Studies and Research on Fasting and Cancer:

Numerous research and anecdotal stories have demonstrated the potential benefits of fasting for cancer patients. Here are some noteworthy examples:

1. Studies on Fasting and Chemotherapy:

Research has revealed that shortterm fasting can improve chemotherapy efficacy by sensitizing cancer cells to treatment while sparing normal cells. Fasting before chemotherapy has been shown to minimize side effects and improve treatment success.

2. Clinical Trials of FastingMimicking Diet:

Clinical investigations on the fastingmimicking diet (FMD) have shown that it can lower cancer risk factors and improve cancer treatment. Participants who completed the FMD demonstrated lower levels of IGF1, better metabolic health, and greater immunological function.

3. Patient testimonials:

Many cancer patients have reported beneficial results from fasting, such as increased energy, fewer treatment side effects, and better general wellbeing. While individual experiences differ, these testimonials demonstrate the potential of fasting as a supportive therapy.

CHAPTER 9

Holistic Lifestyle Changes

Adopting a holistic lifestyle can be revolutionary on the path to cancer recovery and overall wellbeing. Holistic techniques include a variety of approaches that address the physical, emotional, mental, and spiritual components of wellness. This chapter looks at how to incorporate holistic practices into daily living, establish a supportive environment, and devise longterm wellness initiatives.

Integrating Holistic Practices Into Daily Life
Integrating holistic practices into daily life entails establishing routines and habits that promote balance and harmony in the body, mind, and spirit. These habits not only help in cancer recovery, but also improve general quality of life.

1. Mindfulness and meditation:
Mindfulness and meditation are effective strategies for stress reduction, mental clarity, and emotional resilience. Regular practice can help cancer patients cope with anxiety, despair, and the emotional problems of their diagnosis and treatment.
Mindfulness is the practice of being fully present in the moment, paying attention to thoughts, feelings, and sensations without judgment. It can be done by doing mindful breathing, mindful eating, or simply paying attention to regular routines.
Meditation entails allotted time for calm meditation and mental concentration. Guided meditation, mantra meditation, and lovingkindness meditation can all bring significant advantages. Even a few minutes of meditation every day can significantly improve one's mental and emotional wellbeing.

2. Yoga & Gentle Exercise:
Physical activity is essential for preserving strength, flexibility, and good health. Yoga, tai chi, and other gentle exercises are especially beneficial to cancer patients because they combine physical activity with awareness and breath control.

Yoga improves flexibility, strength, and balance while also encouraging relaxation and stress reduction. Hatha, Vinyasa, and Restorative yoga provide varied levels of intensity and can be tailored to individual needs.

Tai Chi is a martial technique that emphasizes slow, deliberate motions and deep breathing. It promotes balance, coordination, and mental focus, making it an ideal practice for cancer patients.

Walking and Light Cardio: Simple exercises such as walking, swimming, or light cycling can enhance cardiovascular health, mood, and energy levels. Regular, moderate exercise strengthens the immune system and promotes healing.

3. Nutritional balance and hydration

Proper nutrition is essential for overall health. A wellbalanced plantbased diet rich in fruits, vegetables, whole grains, nuts, and seeds delivers critical nutrients while also supporting the body's natural healing processes.

AntiInflammatory Foods: Consuming foods with antiinflammatory characteristics, such as turmeric, ginger, green leafy vegetables, and berries, can help reduce chronic inflammation and improve overall health.

Hydration: Proper hydration is required for detoxification, digestion, and cellular function. Drinking plenty of water and herbal teas throughout the day helps you stay hydrated and promotes general wellbeing.

4. Sleep and rest:

Good sleep is essential for both physical and emotional recuperation. During sleep, the body heals tissues, consolidates memories, and regulates hormone levels. Inadequate sleep can impair the immune system and worsen stress.

Sleep Hygiene: Establishing a consistent sleep schedule, maintaining a pleasant sleep environment, and avoiding stimulants such as caffeine and electronic devices before bedtime can all help to enhance sleep quality.

Rest and Relaxation: Including intervals of rest and relaxation in your daily routine helps reduce stress and promotes healing. Reading, listening to music, and spending time in nature can all help you feel better.

5. Emotional and spiritual support:

Emotional and spiritual wellbeing are essential for holistic health. Addressing emotional needs and developing a sense of purpose and connection can improve resilience and general wellbeing.

Counseling and Therapy: Professional counseling or therapy can help patients manage the emotional challenges of cancer. Cognitivebehavioral therapy (CBT), art therapy, and support groups can all provide coping methods and emotional comfort.

Spiritual Practices: Praying, meditating, or joining a church community can bring consolation, hope, and a sense of purpose. Spirituality can provide a significant source of strength and resilience during difficult circumstances.

Creating a Supportive Environment

A supportive atmosphere is essential for promoting overall health and wellbeing. This encompasses both the physical environment and the social and emotional atmosphere.

1. A Healthy Home Environment:

Creating a healthy home environment entails reducing contaminants, maintaining cleanliness, and cultivating a location that fosters relaxation and wellbeing.

Air Quality: Improving indoor air quality with air purifiers, ventilation, and houseplants can help to limit exposure to pollutants and allergies.

NonToxic Products: Using natural, nontoxic cleaning and personal care products helps limit the body's exposure to chemicals. Avoiding synthetic scents, pesticides, and harsh chemicals promotes a better living environment.

ClutterFree Spaces: Keeping your home clean and tidy might help you relax and feel less stressed. Creating separate rooms for relaxation, meditation, and hobbies can improve overall wellbeing.

2. Social Support Networks:

Strong social support networks offer emotional support, practical help, and a sense of belonging. Building and sustaining strong relationships is critical for overall wellness.

Family and Friends: Maintaining contact with family and friends who can provide emotional support, companionship, and encouragement is essential. Open talking and discussing emotions can help to develop relationships and bring relief.

Support Groups: Joining support groups for cancer patients and survivors can provide a sense of community and understanding. These organizations give a forum for sharing experiences, gaining insights, and receiving encouragement from others facing similar issues.

Professional Support: Speaking with healthcare experts, counselors, and holistic practitioners who understand and support holistic approaches to health can provide helpful advice and support.

3. Work/Life Balance:

Achieving a healthy worklife balance is critical for stress reduction and improved general wellbeing. This includes establishing boundaries, prioritizing selfcare, and seeking contentment in both work and personal life.

Time Management: Effective time management practices, such as prioritizing activities, delegating them, and scheduling frequent breaks, can help to minimize stress and prevent burnout.

SelfCare Practices: Including selfcare activities like exercise, hobbies, and relaxation techniques in daily routines promotes balance and wellbeing.

Flexibility and Adaptability: Being adaptable to shifting situations and health demands is critical. This could include rearranging work hours, requesting accommodations, or investigating alternative job opportunities.

LongTerm Wellness Strategies

Longterm wellness initiatives aim to maintain health and wellbeing across time. These tactics entail making consistent, conscious decisions that promote overall health.

1. Continuous Learning and Adaptation:

Adopting an attitude of constant learning and adaptability is essential for longterm wellness. Staying up to date on current breakthroughs in holistic health, nutrition, and cancer care allows people to make more educated decisions.

Educational Resources: Reading books, articles, attending workshops, and taking online courses on holistic health and wellness can help you gain new insights and solutions.

Professional Guidance: Consulting with healthcare professionals, holistic practitioners, and nutritionists can provide individualized guidance and support for your ongoing health requirements.

2. Preventative Health Measures:

Preventive health activities are critical to lowering the chance of cancer recurrence and improving overall health. Regular checkups, screenings, and preventive health habits can aid in the early detection and resolution of any disorders.

Routine Health Screenings: Regular screenings, such as mammograms, colonoscopies, and blood tests, can aid in the early detection of cancer and other health concerns.

Healthy Lifestyle Choices: Making and sticking to healthy lifestyle choices including eating a balanced diet, exercising regularly, and managing stress promotes longterm health and lowers the risk of chronic diseases.

3. Emotional Resilience & Mental Health:

Longterm wellbeing relies heavily on emotional resilience and mental health maintenance. Developing coping methods and emotional abilities helps you manage life's problems more easily.

Stress Management Techniques: Including stress management techniques like mindfulness, meditation, deep breathing exercises, and relaxation techniques in your everyday routines can help reduce stress and promote emotional balance.

Emotional Awareness: Developing emotional awareness and selfcompassion entails identifying and honoring one's emotions without passing judgment. Gratitude, journaling, and artistic expression can all help you feel better emotionally.

Professional help: Seeking continuing help from mental health specialists, such as therapists or counselors, can provide invaluable tools and insights into sustaining emotional health and resilience.

4. Spiritual development and fulfillment:

Spiritual development and fulfillment promote a sense of purpose and overall wellbeing. Spiritual practices and personal beliefs can bring solace, insight, and a stronger connection to life.

Regular Practice: Developing a consistent spiritual practice, such as prayer, meditation, or attendance at religious services, promotes spiritual growth and fulfillment.

Community Involvement: Participating in spiritual or faithbased communities gives you a sense of belonging and support. These communities frequently provide chances for service, friendship, and personal development.

Personal Exploration: Investigating and deepening personal ideas and ideals can lead to improved selfawareness and fulfillment. Reading spiritual books, going on retreats, and engaging in contemplative practices can all help with this journey.

5. Creating Joy and Meaning:

Finding joy and meaning in daily life is critical for longterm wellbeing. Pursuing passions, hobbies, and activities that bring satisfaction and fulfillment improves overall quality of life.

Pursuing Passions: Participating in activities that bring delight and enthusiasm, such as gardening.

Painting, writing, and playing music all bring a sense of purpose and fulfillment.

Social Engagement: Maintaining social activity and developing meaningful relationships improves emotional wellbeing and fosters a sense of community.

Volunteering and Service: Volunteering and giving back to the community promotes a sense of purpose and belonging. Acts of service can be extremely fulfilling and offer chances for personal development.

6. Monitoring and adjusting health practices

Regularly evaluating and updating health practices ensures that they adapt to changing demands and situations. Being proactive and attentive to health changes promotes longterm wellbeing.

Health Tracking: Monitoring health indicators like weight, blood pressure, and energy levels can help you uncover patterns and areas for improvement. Journaling about your food, exercise routine, and emotional wellbeing might yield useful insights.

Adjusting Strategies: Being willing to modify health strategies in response to new information or changing demands is critical. Flexibility and adaptation are essential for sustaining longterm wellness.

CHAPTER 10

Emotional and Mental Wellbeing

Emotional and mental wellbeing are important aspects of overall health, especially for cancer patients. This chapter discusses the mindbody link, approaches for obtaining emotional balance, and the value of support systems and counseling.

THE MINDBODY CONNECTION

The mindbody connection acknowledges that our thoughts, emotions, and physical health are inextricably linked. Understanding and cultivating this relationship has a substantial impact on cancer healing and overall wellbeing.

1. Psychoneuroimmunology:

Psychoneuroimmunology (PNI) is the study of how psychological variables such as stress, emotions, and mental states influence the immune system and overall health. According to PNI research, continuous stress and negative emotions can impair the immune system, making the body more prone to sickness, including cancer.

Stress and Immunity: Chronic stress causes the release of stress hormones such as cortisol, which can reduce immune function and increase inflammation. This reduced immune response may impair the body's capacity to combat cancer cells.

Positive Emotions and Healing: Studies have shown that positive emotions like joy, love, and gratitude improve immune function and promote healing. Mindfulness, meditation, and social connection are examples of practices that promote pleasant feelings and can help cancer patients recover.

2. Role of Stress:

Stress is a natural reaction to difficult events, but it can be harmful to one's health if it is not controlled correctly. Stress in cancer patients can worsen symptoms, diminish treatment efficacy, and impair overall health.

Physical Signs of Stress: Stress can cause weariness, headaches, muscle tension, and digestive problems. It might also cause sleep difficulties and reduced immunity.

Emotional Effects of Stress: Stress can produce anxiety, despair, impatience, and feelings of overload. These emotional states can influence decisionmaking, relationships, and the ability to deal with cancer therapy.

Stress Management: Effective stress management practices, such as mindfulness, relaxation exercises, physical activity, and hobbies, can help to reduce the detrimental effects of stress on health.

3. Mindfulness & Mental Health:

Mindfulness is the discipline of being fully present in the moment, observing thoughts, emotions, and sensations without judgment. Mindfulness has been demonstrated to lower stress, increase mental clarity, and improve emotional regulation.

Mindfulness Practices: Common mindfulness techniques include mindful breathing, body scanning, and mindful meditation. These techniques can be readily incorporated into everyday routines to improve mental and emotional health.

Benefits for Cancer Patients: Mindfulness can help cancer patients cope with treatmentrelated stress, reduce anxiety and depression, improve sleep, and improve overall quality of life.

Techniques for Emotional Balance

Achieving emotional balance entails implementing habits and approaches that promote mental and emotional wellness. These approaches can help cancer patients deal with the emotional problems of their diagnosis and treatment.

1. Cognitive Behavior Therapy (CBT):

CognitiveBehavioral Therapy (CBT) is an organized, timelimited treatment that aims to uncover and change problematic thought patterns and behaviors. CBT has been demonstrated to be useful for anxiety, depression, and stressrelated disorders.

CBT strategies: CBT strategies include cognitive restructuring, which involves challenging and reframing negative thinking, as well as behavioral activation, which encourages participation in positive activities. These approaches can assist cancer patients in managing emotional distress and improving coping abilities.

Benefits for Cancer Patients: Cognitive behavioural therapy (CBT) can help cancer patients reduce anxiety and depression, increase emotional resilience, and improve their overall quality of life. It offers practical strategies for dealing with stress and emotional issues.

2. Relaxation techniques:

Relaxation practices improve both physical and mental relaxation, lowering stress and increasing emotional wellbeing. These procedures can be simply applied at home or in conjunction with other therapy.

Deep Breathing: Deep breathing techniques, such diaphragmatic breathing or the 478 technique, can help the body relax and reduce tension.

Progressive Muscle Relaxation (PMR): PMR consists of tensing and releasing various muscle groups in the body to promote physical relaxation and reduce muscle tension.

Guided Imagery: Guided imagery entails envisioning relaxing and positive pictures, such as a tranquil beach or a serene forest. This practice can help with stress reduction, mood enhancement, and emotional wellbeing.

3. Mindful Meditation:

Mindfulness meditation entails focusing attention on the present moment while monitoring thoughts and feelings without judgment. This technique can reduce stress, improve emotional regulation, and boost general wellbeing.

Breathing Meditation: Concentrating on the breath as it flows in and out can help to focus and relax the mind. This simple practice can be performed anywhere and at any time.

Body Scan Meditation: This technique is systematically focusing on various regions of the body, from head to toe, and noting sensations without judgment. It encourages physical relaxation and bodily awareness.

LovingKindness Meditation: This practice focuses on developing sentiments of love and compassion for oneself and others. It can boost pleasant feelings, reduce stress, and promote emotional health.

4. Emotional expression and journaling:

Expressing feelings through writing or other kinds of creative expression can bring emotional relief while also improving mental clarity. Journaling, in particular, is an extremely effective method for processing thoughts and emotions.

Reflective Journaling: Writing about daily experiences, emotions, and thoughts might help cancer patients understand their emotional condition and recognize patterns. Reflective journaling encourages selfawareness and emotional processing.

Gratitude Journaling: Focusing on the positive parts of life and writing down what one is grateful for can boost positive emotions and improve overall wellbeing.

Art and Music Therapy: Creative activities like drawing, painting, or performing music can provide a nonverbal avenue for emotional expression while also promoting relaxation.

5. Physical activity:

Physical activity improves not just physical health but also mental and emotional wellbeing. Exercise can help with stress reduction, mood improvement, and general quality of life.

Aerobic Exercise: Walking, jogging, swimming, or dancing can increase endorphins, lower stress, and enhance mood.

Strength Training: Exercises like lifting weights or utilizing resistance bands can help you gain physical strength, confidence, and emotional wellbeing.

MindBody Exercises: Yoga, tai chi, and qigong incorporate physical movement, awareness, and breath control to promote relaxation and emotional balance.

SUPPORT SYSTEMS AND COUNSELING

Cancer sufferers benefit greatly from support systems and counseling. These materials can help with coping skills, minimize isolation, and increase general wellbeing.

1. Family and friends:

For many cancer patients, family and friends are their primary sources of emotional support. Strong social relationships can provide emotional support, encouragement, and practical assistance.

Open Communication: Communicating openly and honestly with loved ones can help to develop relationships and bring emotional relief. Sharing feelings and experiences can lead to greater understanding and support.

Supportive Activities: Participating in activities with family and friends, such as social events, outings, or hobbies, can provide beneficial distractions while also improving mental health.

Seeking Help: Encourage family and friends to seek cancer support and knowledge so that they can better support the sufferer. Support groups and counseling for caregivers can also be helpful.

2. Support Groups:

Support groups offer cancer patients a secure area to connect with others who are facing similar struggles. These groups provide emotional support, practical assistance, and a sense of community.

Benefits of Support Groups: Joining a support group can help you feel less isolated, improve your coping abilities, and learn more about cancer treatment and management.

Types of Support Groups: Support groups can be organized by cancer kind, treatment stage, or demographic (e.g., young people, women, males). Online support groups and forums provide increased flexibility and accessibility.

Finding Support Groups: Healthcare practitioners, cancer centers, and organizations like the American Cancer Society can help you find local and online support groups.

3. Professional counseling and therapy:

Professional counseling and therapy offer cancer patients an organized and supportive setting in which to examine and resolve their emotional concerns. Therapists can provide evidencebased treatments as well as personalized help.

Individual Therapy: Oneonone sessions with a certified therapist can help cancer patients deal with anxiety, despair, trauma, and other emotional concerns. Therapists can provide coping skills and emotional support that are suited to each individual's requirements.

Group Therapy: Multiple patients collaborate with a therapist in a group environment. It combines the benefits of peer support and shared experiences with expert coaching.

Family Therapy: The patient and their family members collaborate with a therapist to address relational and emotional concerns. It can increase communication, develop family relationships, and boost group coping.

4. Spiritual and Faithbased Support:

Spiritual and faithbased support can give many cancer sufferers peace, hope, and a sense of purpose. Engaging in spiritual practices and engaging with faith communities can help you feel better emotionally.

Spiritual Counseling: Spiritual counselors, such as chaplains or religious leaders, can provide direction, support, and prayer based on the patient's spiritual beliefs and needs.

Faith Communities: Joining a faith community provides a sense of belonging and support. Religious services, prayer groups, and spiritual retreats can provide support and connection.

Personal Spiritual Practices: Prayer, meditation, and reading spiritual materials can bring comfort and strength. These activities can be implemented into everyday routines to provide continual support.

5. Holistic and Integrated Therapies:

Holistic and integrative therapies, such as acupuncture, massage therapy, and energy healing, can supplement conventional medical treatments and promote emotional wellbeing.

Acupuncture: Acupuncture is the process of inserting thin needles into certain places on the body to promote balance and healing. It can reduce stress, relieve pain, and improve general health.

Massage treatment: Massage treatment can help relieve muscle tension, promote relaxation, and boost emotional wellbeing. Swedish massage, deep tissue massage, and aromatherapy massage are all techniques that can be adjusted to individual needs.

Energy Healing: Practices like Reiki and healing touch manipulate energy fields to promote balance and healing. These therapies can help with stress management, relaxation, and emotional wellbeing.

6. Education Resources:

Access to educational resources provides cancer patients with awareness of their diagnosis, treatment alternatives, and coping skills. Informed patients can make better decisions and control their health.

Books and Articles: Reading about cancer, holistic health, and emotional wellbeing can bring useful information and insights. Recommended readings include writings by healthcare experts, survivors, and holistic practitioners.

Workshops and Seminars: Attending workshops and seminars on cancer care, stress management, and holistic health can provide useful information and support. Many cancer facilities and organizations host educational activities.

Online Resources: Websites, webinars, and virtual support groups offer easily available information and support. The National Cancer Institute, the American Cancer Society, and holistic health websites are all reputable sources.

CHAPTER 11

Recipes and Menu Plans

Dr. Sebi's approach to healing and cancer recovery is based mostly on nutrition. This chapter delves further into alkaline recipes, sample meal plans, and suggestions for making therapeutic foods. These tools are intended to assist people incorporate Dr. Sebi's dietary ideas into their daily lives, thereby improving their general health and wellbeing.

INTRODUCTION TO ALKALINE RECIPES

The alkaline diet is important to Dr. Sebi's nutritional philosophy, focusing on natural, plantbased foods that foster an alkaline internal environment. This section discusses the basics of alkaline recipes and their benefits for cancer prevention and recovery.

1. Understanding alkaline foods:

 Alkaline meals are those that, when metabolized, leave an alkaline residue in the body, which helps to balance the pH levels. Dr. Sebi's diet prioritizes these foods in order to preserve good health and prevent disease.

 Benefits for Cancer Patients: Consuming an alkaline diet can help reduce inflammation, boost immune function, and create an internal environment that is less conducive to cancer cell proliferation. This diet also encourages detoxification, which is essential for people receiving cancer treatments.

2. Key Alkaline Foods:

 Vegetables: Leafy greens (kale, spinach, collard greens), cucumbers, bell peppers, zucchini, and broccoli are all extremely alkaline and high in important elements.

 Fruits: Berries (blueberries, strawberries), citrus fruits (lemons, limes), melons, and avocados are alkalineforming and provide essential vitamins, antioxidants, and water.

 Nuts and Seeds: Almonds, flaxseeds, chia seeds, and pumpkin seeds are high in nutrients and alkaline in nature, providing healthy fats, protein, and fiber.

Grains: Quinoa, amaranth, and wild rice are some of the few grains permitted in Dr. Sebi's diet due to their alkaline qualities and nutritional value.

Herbs and Spices: Basil, cilantro, oregano, thyme, and ginger are alkaline, but they also have medicinal characteristics that promote health and healing.

3. Avoid Acidic Foods:

Acidic diets create an interior milieu that promotes inflammation and sickness. Dr. Sebi's diet recommends avoiding certain foods in order to preserve an alkaline balance.

Common Acidic Foods: Processed foods, refined sugars, dairy products, red meat, and most cereals (such as wheat and corn) are all acidic. Avoiding these foods reduces the body's acid load and promotes general wellness.

4. Balancing Meal:

Balancing meals with a variety of alkaline foods guarantees that the diet is nutrientdense and beneficial to health. Each meal should contain a variety of vegetables, fruits, nuts, seeds, and allowed grains.

Meal Composition: Aim for a plate that contains at least 7080% alkalineforming meals, with the rest neutral or slightly acidic items. This equilibrium helps to maintain normal pH levels and promotes general health.

SAMPLE MEAL PLANS

Creating regular meal planning can help people follow Dr. Sebi's dietary advice and make it easier to incorporate alkaline foods into their diets. This section includes sample weeklong meal plans that feature a variety of delicious and nutritionally balanced meals.

1. Breakfast:

Day 1:

Green Smoothie

Combine kale, spinach, cucumber, apple, lemon juice, and a handful of almonds for a nutritious start to the day.

Day 2:

Quinoa Porridge Cook quinoa in almond milk, add fresh berries, then top with chia seeds and agave honey.

Day 3:

Avocado Toast: Mash avocado on sprouted grain bread, then top with sliced tomatoes and a sprinkling of sea salt and pepper.

Day 4:

Fresh Fruit Salad Mix together berries, melons, and citrus fruits, then top with a handful of pumpkin seeds.

Day 5: Chia Seed Pudding Soak chia seeds in almond milk overnight, then combine with a touch of vanilla essence and top with sliced bananas and almonds.

Day 6:

Vegetable Omelette Make an omelette using spinach, bell peppers, onions, and tomatoes, and use chickpea flour as the basis.

Day 7:

Smoothie Bowl Combine frozen berries, banana, and almond milk; top with sliced fruit, almonds, and seeds.

2. Lunch:

Day 1: Quinoa Salad: Combine cooked quinoa, chopped cucumbers, bell peppers, cherry tomatoes, red onions, and a lemonolive oil dressing.

Day 2:

Vegetable StirFry: Sauté broccoli, zucchini, bell peppers, and snap peas in coconut oil with ginger and garlic before serving over wild rice.

Day 3:

Stuffed Bell Peppers: Fill bell peppers with quinoa, black beans, corn, and spices, then bake until soft.

Day 4: Chickpea Salad Wrap Mix chickpeas, chopped cucumbers, tomatoes, red onions, and avocado in a lettuce wrap.

Day 5: Roasted Vegetable Bowl Roast a variety of root vegetables (carrots, sweet potatoes, and beets) and serve with tahini dressing.

Day 6:

Zucchini Noodles Mix spiralized zucchini with homemade tomato basil sauce and top with nutritional yeast.

Day 7: Lentil Soup Make a hearty soup with lentils, carrots, celery, onions, and spinach in vegetable broth.

3. Dinner:

Day 1:

Grilled Portobello Mushrooms: Marinate portobello mushrooms in balsamic vinegar and herbs, then grill and serve with sautéed spinach.

Day 2:

Eggplant Parmesan: Layer eggplant slices with marinara sauce and nutritional yeast, then bake until golden brown.

Day 3: packed Squash Roasted acorn squash halves packed with wild rice, cranberries, walnuts, and spices.

Day 4:

Cauliflower Rice Bowl: Sauté riced cauliflower with turmeric, garlic, and a variety of colorful veggies.

Day 5: Vegetable Curry Prepare a vegetable curry using coconut milk, sweet potatoes, bell peppers, and spinach, and serve over quinoa.

Day 6:

Roast spaghetti squash, then top with homemade marinara sauce and fresh basil.

Day 7:

Mushroom Stroganoff Make a creamy stroganoff with mushrooms, onions, and a cashewbased sauce; serve over brown rice.

4. Snack and Beverage:

Alkaline Snacks: Cucumber slices and hummus, raw almonds, mixed berries, avocado slices, and veggie sticks with guacamole.

Beverages: Herbal teas (e.g., ginger, chamomile, peppermint), lemoninfused alkaline water, fresh vegetable juices, and almond milk and fruit smoothies.

Preparing Healing Foods

Proper cooking of alkaline foods improves their therapeutic powers and maximizes nutritional benefits. This section includes recommendations and tips for preparing and cooking dishes in accordance with Dr. Sebi's philosophy.

1. Cooking methods:

Steaming and boiling: These gentle cooking methods conserve nutrients and improve the digestibility of veggies. Steaming is especially helpful for greens, while boiling is ideal for root veggies.

Grilling and Baking: Grilling and baking enhance the flavor of vegetables without the use of excessive oils. Marinating vegetables in herbs and spices before grilling or baking can improve their flavor and nutrients.

Sautéing: Sautéing veggies in healthy oils such as coconut or olive oil is a quick and nutritious meal preparation method. Adding herbs and spices throughout the sautéing process might increase the dish's nutritional value.

Raw Preparation: Consuming raw vegetables and fruits retains their natural enzymes and nutrients. Salads, smoothies, and raw snacks are great ways to include raw foods in your diet.

2. Meal Preparation Tip:

Batch Cooking: Preparing large quantities of grains, legumes, and veggies ahead of time saves time and ensures that nutritious meals are always available. Batch cooking also simplifies meal preparation throughout the week.

Storage: Proper storage of prepared foods is critical for preserving freshness and nutritious content. Refrigerate and freeze meals in sealed containers to ensure they are ready to use.

Meal Planning: Planning meals ahead of time helps to ensure a balanced diet and decreases the risk of eating less healthful foods. A weekly meal plan might help with grocery shopping and meal preparation.

3. Adding Herbs and Spices:

Flavor and Health: Herbs and spices not only enhance the flavor of food, but they also provide significant health benefits. Adding a variety of herbs and spices to foods might boost their therapeutic effects.

Common Herbs and Spices: Dr. Sebi highly recommends basil, oregano, thyme, cilantro, turmeric, ginger, and garlic in his diet. These items can be used in a number of recipes, including salads, soups, and main courses.

Herb Preparation: Fresh herbs are preferred, but dried herbs are also acceptable. Adding herbs near the end of cooking retains their flavor and nutritional value.

4. SuperFoods and Supplements:

Superfoods: Some foods are dubbed "superfoods" because of their high nutrient content and health advantages. Examples include spirulina, chlorella, sea moss, and hemp seeds. These can be added to smoothies, salads, and other foods.

Natural Supplements: While a wellbalanced diet should provide the majority of nutrients, natural supplements can aid with specific deficits. Dr. Sebi recommends supplements such as burdock root, bladderwrack, and sarsaparilla.

CHAPTER 13

Combating Certain Types of Cancer

This chapter focuses on Dr. Sebi's specialized techniques to treat certain forms of cancer, such as breast cancer, prostate cancer, and lung cancer. Each part digs into the unique features of these diseases and provides natural management techniques, with a focus on holistic therapy, plantbased diet, and detoxification.

TAILORED APPROACHES TO BREAST CANCER

Breast cancer is one of the most frequent cancers among women worldwide. It is the development of malignant cells in breast tissue that can be impacted by a number of genetic, hormonal, and environmental variables. Dr. Sebi's approach to breast cancer focuses on building an interior environment that inhibits cancer cell proliferation while promoting overall wellness.

1. Understanding Breast Cancer:

Breast cancer starts in the cells of the breast, usually in the milk ducts or lobule. If not diagnosed and treated promptly, it has the potential to spread to adjacent tissues and other sections of the body.

Risk factors include genetic predisposition (such as BRCA1 and BRCA2 mutations), hormone imbalances, lifestyle choices (diet, physical exercise), and exposure to environmental pollutants.

2. Nutritional Strategy:

Alkaline Diet: Eating more alkalineforming foods helps to maintain a regulated pH in the body, which reduces inflammation and creates an environment less conducive to cancer formation. Leafy greens, cruciferous veggies, berries, and citrus fruits are very nutritious.

Phytoestrogens: Certain plant substances, such as flaxseeds, soy, and legumes, can help regulate hormones by imitating the actions of estrogen. These phytoestrogens may be especially effective in hormonesensitive breast cancers.

AntioxidantRich Foods: Antioxidants shield cells from oxidative damage, which can lead to cancer growth. Antioxidantrich foods include berries, nuts, seeds, and dark leafy greens.

3. Herbal Remedy:

Burdock Root: Burdock root is known for its bloodpurifying characteristics, which can aid in detoxification and immune system support. It is commonly used in teas and supplements.

Red Clover: High in isoflavones, red clover may help regulate hormones and lower the incidence of hormonedependent malignancies. It can be taken as a tea or in supplement form.

Milk Thistle: This herb promotes liver detoxification, which is essential for hormonal balance and overall health. Milk thistle extract can be consumed as a supplement or in tea form.

4. Detoxification and Lifestyle Adjustments:

Regular Detoxification: Regular detoxification helps to eliminate pollutants that can lead to cancer growth. Dr. Sebi suggests drinking herbal teas, fasting, and eating detoxifying foods such as garlic, turmeric, and green vegetables.

Physical Activity: Regular exercise promotes overall health, enhances immunological function, and aids in the maintenance of a healthy weight, which can lower the risk of breast cancer.

Stress Management: Chronic stress can impair the immune system and accelerate cancer progression. Meditation, yoga, and deep breathing techniques are all effective ways to handle stress.

PROSTATE CANCER TREATMENT STRATEGIES

Prostate cancer is the most frequent cancer in men, primarily affecting those over the age of 50. It is the development of cancerous cells in the prostate gland, which can impair urine and sexual function. Dr. Sebi's approach to prostate cancer treatment involves dietary adjustments, herbal medicines, and lifestyle changes that promote prostate health and general wellbeing.

1. Understanding Prostate Cancer:

Prostate cancer occurs in the prostate gland, which produces seminal fluid. It can develop slowly or aggressively, spreading swiftly.

Risk factors include age, family history, race (more common in African American men), diet, and lifestyle.

2. Nutritional Strategy:

PlantBased Diet: A diet high in fruits and vegetables, whole grains, nuts, and seeds promotes prostate health. Foods high in lycopene, such as tomatoes, cruciferous vegetables (broccoli, cauliflower), and berries, have been demonstrated to lessen the incidence of prostate cancer.

Healthy Fats: Flaxseed, chia seeds, and walnuts contain omega3 fatty acids, which can help reduce inflammation and promote prostate health. Avoiding saturated and trans fats is also important.

ZincRich Foods: Zinc is beneficial to prostate health. Foods rich in zinc include pumpkin seeds, almonds, and chickpeas.

3. Herbal Remedy:

Saw Palmetto: Saw palmetto is known for its prostate health advantages, including the ability to alleviate symptoms of an enlarged prostate and perhaps anticancer qualities.

Nettle Root: This herb promotes urinary health and may help ease symptoms of prostate enlargement.

Pygeum: Made from the bark of the African cherry tree, pygeum is used to treat prostate and urinary issues.

4. Detoxification and Lifestyle Adjustments:

Regular Detoxification: Detoxifying the body helps remove toxic compounds that can cause prostate problems. It is advisable to drink herbal teas, fast, and consume cleansing meals.

Physical Activity: Regular exercise improves general health, helps maintain a healthy weight, and may lower the risk of prostate cancer.

Stress Management: Meditation, yoga, and relaxation techniques can help improve immune function and overall wellbeing.

MANAGE LUNG CANCER NATURALLY.

Lung cancer is one of the main causes of cancerrelated deaths globally, primarily affecting those who have smoked, but nonsmokers can also acquire lung cancer. Dr. Sebi's approach to lung cancer treatment includes dietary treatments, herbal therapies, and lifestyle changes that promote lung health and overall recovery.

1. Understanding Lung Cancer:

Lung cancer develops in the lungs and spreads throughout the body. The two primary forms are nonsmall cell lung cancer (NSCLC) and small cell lung cancer (SCLC).

Risk factors include smoking, secondhand smoke exposure, carcinogen exposure (e.g., asbestos and radon), and genetic susceptibility.

2. Nutritional Strategy:

AntiInflammatory Diet: An antiinflammatory diet lowers inflammation and improves immunological function. Turmeric, ginger, garlic, and green leafy vegetables are quite healthy.

AntioxidantRich Foods: Antioxidants help prevent lung cell damage. Berries, nuts, seeds, and dark leafy greens are antioxidantrich foods.

Hydration: Staying hydrated promotes lung health and aids the body's detoxification process. Drinking plenty of water, herbal teas, and eating waterrich foods such as cucumbers and melons is recommended.

3. Herbal Remedy:

Lungwort: Lungwort is wellknown for its respiratory effects, and it can calm and mend lung tissue. It can be taken as a tea or in supplement form.

Licorice Root: This herb has antiinflammatory and immuneboosting characteristics, which make it good for lung health. Licorice root can be consumed as tea or in supplement form.

Mullein: Mullein is wellknown for its potential to promote lung health and mucus clearance. It can be drunk as tea or used in herbal remedies.

4. Detoxification and Lifestyle Adjustments:

Regular Detoxification: Detoxifying the body helps to eliminate toxic compounds that can contribute to lung cancer. It is advisable to drink herbal teas, fast, and consume cleansing meals.

Smoking Cessation: Quitting smoking is essential for lung cancer prevention and treatment. Individuals can quit smoking through support programs, counseling, and natural cures.

Breathing Exercises: Breathing exercises can help increase lung capacity and function. Diaphragmatic breathing, pursedlip breathing, and yoga breathing exercises are all effective.

5. Environmental considerations:

Air Quality: Having clean air in your home and workplace is critical for lung health. Using air purifiers, avoiding pollutants, and spending time in natural, unpolluted areas can all assist.

Avoiding Carcinogens: Limiting exposure to known carcinogens such as asbestos, radon, and industrial pollutants is critical for preventing lung cancer.

CHAPTER 14

Supplemental Practices

This chapter delves into other practices that augment Dr. Sebi's comprehensive approach to cancer prevention and recovery. These practices include yoga, meditation, acupuncture, massage, and other complementary therapies. Each practice has distinct benefits for physical, mental, and emotional wellbeing, increasing the overall efficacy of a holistic healing process.

Integrating Yoga and Meditation
Yoga and meditation are ancient techniques that encourage balance in the body, mind, and spirit. They provide several benefits to cancer patients, including less stress, higher sleep quality, improved immunological function, and a stronger sense of wellbeing. Integrating yoga and meditation into a holistic healing program can be extremely beneficial during cancer treatment and recovery.

1. Yoga For Cancer Patients:
soft Movement: Yoga positions can be adapted to accommodate cancer patients by emphasizing soft movements that improve flexibility, strength, and balance.
Breath Awareness: Pranayama, or yogic breathing methods, serve to relax the mind, reduce tension, and promote oxygenation in the body's tissues. Deep, diaphragmatic breathing promotes relaxation and overall wellbeing.
Mindfulness: Practicing mindfulness during yoga sessions improves presentmoment awareness and acceptance of one's bodily and emotional states. This can be especially helpful in reducing worry and panic linked with cancer diagnosis and treatment.

2. Meditation For Cancer Patients:
Stress Reduction: Meditation techniques including mindfulness meditation, guided imagery, and lovingkindness meditation enhance relaxation while reducing the physiological consequences of stress

on the body. Regular meditation practice can assist to reduce anxiety, depression, and emotional suffering.

Pain Management: Mindfulnessbased pain management strategies help people build a new relationship with suffering, promoting more acceptance and resilience. Meditation can help with pain perception and coping methods.

Emotional Healing: Meditation creates a safe environment for processing tough emotions including loss, rage, and uncertainty. Individuals can grow emotional resilience and find serenity in the face of cancer hardships by practicing compassionate selfawareness.

3. How to Integrate Yoga and Meditation into Your Daily Life:

Consistency: To fully benefit from yoga and meditation, it is essential to establish a regular practice. Begin with brief sessions and progressively increase the duration and intensity as your comfort and confidence improve.

Adaptation: Customize yoga poses and meditation practices to meet your specific demands and physical constraints. Seek guidance from competent educators who are familiar with working with cancer patients.

Community Support: Attending yoga sessions or meditation groups intended exclusively for cancer patients promotes a sense of community and connection with others who understand and empathize with your situation.

Benefits of Acupuncture and Massage

Acupuncture and massage treatment are traditional medicinal techniques that promote relaxation, pain alleviation, and overall health. These techniques boost the body's natural healing mechanisms, improve circulation, and promote emotional wellbeing. Acupuncture and massage, when combined with a comprehensive cancer care plan, can supplement conventional treatments while also improving quality of life.

1. Acupuncture for Cancer Patients:

Pain Management: Acupuncture effectively relieves cancerrelated pain, such as neuropathic pain, musculoskeletal pain, and treatmentrelated adverse effects. Acupuncture regulates pain signals and stimulates the release of endorphins, the body's natural painrelieving compounds.

Nausea and Vomiting: Studies have shown that acupuncture can lessen chemotherapyinduced nausea and vomiting, enhancing treatment tolerance and quality of life for cancer patients. It may also help with other treatmentrelated symptoms, like exhaustion, sleeplessness, and hot flashes.

Immune Support: Acupuncture boosts the immune system by modulating immunological responses and improving the body's ability to combat infection and disease. This immuneboosting effect may be especially advantageous for people undergoing cancer treatment.

2. Massage Treatment for Cancer Patients:

Pain Relief: Massage treatment relieves muscle tension, reduces pain, and improves range of motion in cancer patients. Swedish massage, deep tissue massage, and lymphatic drainage massage are all techniques that target specific areas of discomfort while promoting relaxation.

Stress Reduction: Massage therapy causes profound relaxation, which calms the nervous system and lowers stress chemicals such as cortisol. Regular massage treatments can help with anxiety, despair, and emotional discomfort related to cancer diagnosis and treatment.

Improved Sleep Quality: Massage relaxes and improves sleep quality, which is critical for general health and healing. Cancer patients frequently have sleep problems due to pain, worry, and medication side effects. Massage therapy can assist regulate sleep patterns and promote restful sleep.

3. Safety Considerations:

Consultation with Healthcare professionals: Before beginning acupuncture or massage therapy, cancer patients should consult with their healthcare professionals to confirm that these treatments are safe and appropriate for their medical condition and treatment plan.

Experienced Practitioners: Select licensed acupuncturists and qualified massage therapists who have already worked with cancer patients. They should understand the contraindications, precautions, and suitable approaches for people undergoing cancer therapy.

Communication and Feedback: Talk freely with your acupuncturist or massage therapist about your symptoms, treatment goals, and degree of comfort throughout sessions. Give input on the pressure, intensity, and areas of concern to promote a happy and helpful experience.

ADDITIONAL COMPLEMENTARY THERAPIES

Yoga, meditation, acupuncture, and massage are just a few of the complementary therapies that can help cancer patients recuperate. These therapies cover a wide range of methods, such as energy healing, aromatherapy, art therapy, and music therapy. Each provides distinct physical, emotional, and spiritual advantages, improving cancer patients' entire quality of life.

1. Energy Healing:

Reiki: Reiki is a Japanese energy healing therapy that helps with relaxation, stress reduction, and emotional balance. Reiki practitioners use universal life force energy to help the body's natural healing process.

Healing Touch: This mild, noninvasive energy therapy promotes relaxation, pain alleviation, and emotional wellbeing. Practitioners utilize light touch or nearbody procedures to restore the body's energy field and facilitate healing.

Qi Gong: Qi Gong is a Chinese mindbody exercise that uses gentle movement, breathwork, and visualization to increase vital energy (qi) and promote health and longevity. Qi Gong activities are adaptable for people of various ages and fitness levels.

2. Aromatherapy:

Essential Oils: For millennia, essential oils extracted from plants have been utilized to boost physical and emotional health. Lavender, chamomile, peppermint, and frankincense are some of the most common essential oils used to relieve tension, pain, and induce relaxation.

Diffusion and Topical Application: Essential oils inhaled by diffusion or applied topically can have a therapeutic effect on the body and mind. Aromatherapy massage, baths, and inhalation techniques are popular ways to include essential oils into a holistic therapeutic plan.

3. Art and Music Therapy:

Art Therapy: Art therapy encourages emotional healing and selfdiscovery through creative expressions such as painting, drawing, and sculpting. Art therapy can help cancer patients manage unpleasant emotions, explore their inner world, and feel empowered and selfexpressive. Art therapy sessions are led by qualified therapists who create a secure and supportive environment in which people can engage in the creative process.

Music Therapy: Music therapy harnesses the power of music to alleviate physical, emotional, cognitive, and social issues. Cancer patients can benefit from listening to music, making music, or taking part in guided musicbased activities. Music therapy can help with anxiety, mood, and quality of life throughout cancer treatment and recovery.

4. Nutrition Counseling:

Dietary Guidance: Nutritional counseling offers specialized dietary advice based on the specific needs and preferences of cancer patients. Registered dietitians and nutritionists can assist clients in optimizing their diet to support healing, control treatment side effects, and promote general wellbeing.

Supplement Recommendations: Nutritional counselors may suggest dietary supplements or herbal therapies to address specific nutritional deficits or improve immune function. These supplements should be used in conjunction with a healthy diet and under the supervision of a medical professional.

5. Mind/Body Practices:

Tai Chi: Tai Chi is a peaceful mindbody workout that involves flowing movements, deep breathing, and awareness. It increases relaxation, balance, and flexibility while also improving mental clarity and emotional wellbeing.

Guided Imagery: This technique involves using the imagination to generate positive mental images that promote relaxation, healing, and wellbeing. Cancer sufferers can utilize guided imagery techniques to imagine themselves as healthy, strong, and diseasefree.

INTEGRATING SUPPLEMENTAL PRACTICES INTO CANCER CARE

Integrating supplementary practices into cancer care necessitates a comprehensive, patientcentered strategy that takes into account each individual's specific requirements, preferences, and treatment goals. Here are some important considerations for implementing these approaches into a complete cancer treatment plan:

1. The Collaborative Care Team:

Communication: Communicate openly with all members of the healthcare team, including oncologists, nurses, and supplementary healthcare providers. Share information about the supplemental practices you're contemplating, as well as how they'll fit into your overall treatment strategy.

Coordination: Make sure that every part of your cancer treatment is coordinated and complementary. Your healthcare practitioners should collaborate to develop a comprehensive treatment plan that meets your physical, emotional, and spiritual needs.

2. Informed DecisionMaking: Education: Learn about available supplemental practices, including their benefits and hazards. To make informed selections about which techniques are best for you, consult respected websites, publications, and healthcare specialists.

Personalization: Select supplemental practices that are consistent with your values, preferences, and beliefs. What works for one person may not work for another, so tailor your approach to cancer care to your specific requirements and circumstances.

3. Safety and Monitoring: Consultation: Before beginning any new supplemental practice, consult with your healthcare practitioner to confirm it is safe and appropriate based on your medical history and treatment plan. Certain techniques may have contraindications or interfere with specific drugs.

Monitoring: Track your progress and response to additional practices over time. Keep track of any changes in symptoms, side effects, or overall health and share this information with your healthcare provider.

4. Integration into Daily Life: Consistency: Integrate supplemental techniques into your daily routine to ensure longterm effectiveness. Whether it's making time for yoga and meditation every morning or arranging regular acupuncture or massage appointments, consistency is essential for reaping the full benefits of these disciplines.

Flexibility: Be versatile when it comes to supplemental practices. Life can be unexpected, especially when coping with cancer, so be prepared to adapt your schedule as necessary to meet changes in your health or circumstances.

CHAPTER 15

Future Directions in Natural Healing

In this final chapter, we look at the future of natural health, namely in cancer therapy and holistic wellness. As we move ahead, we look at breakthroughs in holistic cancer treatments, Dr. Sebi's lasting impact on modern medicine, and the continued quest of natural healing.

ADVANCES IN HOLISTIC CANCER TREATMENTS

Holistic cancer treatments use a variety of approaches to address the physical, emotional, and spiritual components of healing. As our understanding of cancer biology and integrative medicine progresses, some promising developments in holistic cancer care emerge.

1. Personalized Medicine: Genomic Profiling: Advances in genomic sequencing technologies allow researchers to detect genetic alterations and molecular biomarkers linked to certain cancer types. This enables individualized treatment approaches that are matched to each individual's unique genetic profile, thereby improving therapeutic efficacy and reducing side effects.

Target Therapies: Targeted therapies preferentially target cancer cells based on their molecular properties, leaving normal cells unaffected. These medicines, which may include monoclonal antibodies, small molecule inhibitors, and immunotherapies, have transformed cancer treatment by providing more specific and effective choices with less systemic adverse effects.

2. Immunotherapy: Immune Checkpoint Inhibitors: Immunotherapy medications use the immune system to target and kill cancer cells. These medications activate the body's natural defenses against cancer by disrupting inhibitory pathways that reduce immune responses, resulting in longterm responses and better results in specific cancers.

- CAR TCell Therapy: CAR Tcell therapy includes genetically modifying a patient's immune cells to recognize and destroy cancer cells. This novel technique has demonstrated extraordinary effectiveness in treating specific blood cancers, such as leukemia and lymphoma, and it has promise for other types of cancer as well.

3. Integrative Oncology: Combination Therapies: Integrative oncology integrates traditional cancer treatments with evidencebased complementary therapies to improve outcomes and quality of life for patients. Acupuncture, massage, mindbody practices, dietary counseling, and herbal medicine are a few examples of such therapies.

Clinical Trial: Clinical trials assessing the efficacy and safety of integrative oncology therapies are now underway to investigate their potential benefits in cancer care. By thoroughly researching these medicines, researchers want to incorporate the most successful and evidencebased approaches into standard cancer therapy procedures.

4. MindBody Medicine: Stress Reduction: Mindfulness meditation, yoga, and relaxation activities aid in cancer care by reducing psychological discomfort, strengthening coping abilities, and overall wellbeing. Integrating mindbody practices into cancer treatment programs can help patients manage symptoms, reduce treatmentrelated adverse effects, and improve overall quality of life.

PsychoOncology: Psychooncology focuses on meeting the psychological, social, and emotional needs of cancer patients and their families during the treatment process. Individual counseling, support groups, and expressive therapies are examples of psychosocial interventions that provide emotional support, improve resilience, and help people adjust to living with cancer.

DR. SEBI'S INFLUENCE ON MODERN MEDICINE

Dr. Sebi, a wellknown herbalist and natural healer, has established a lasting legacy in the field of holistic health. His pioneering work on alkaline diets, herbal cures, and detoxification programs has encouraged millions of people all over the world to embrace natural healing and live better lives. Despite confronting skepticism and controversy throughout his life, Dr. Sebi's ideas continue to connect with people looking for alternative methods to health and wellness.

1. Alkaline Diets and PlantBased Nutrition: Dr. Sebi emphasized the need of ingesting alkalineforming foods for optimal health and illness prevention. His guidelines support scientific data that plantbased diets lessen the risk of chronic diseases like cancer, cardiovascular disease, and diabetes. Dr. Sebi's dietary guidelines are consistent with current recommendations for healthy eating patterns that promote overall wellbeing and disease prevention by encouraging the consumption of fresh fruits, vegetables, nuts, seeds, and whole grains while limiting the intake of processed foods, animal products, and acidic foods.

2. Herbal Remedies and Detoxification: Dr. Sebi's use of herbal remedies and detoxification regimens to cleanse the body and assist natural healing has resonated with those seeking alternative therapies for various health concerns, such as cancer. Traditional herbal therapies have shown potential anticancer benefits in preclinical investigations, yet scientific data need to be established. Research into the mechanisms of action and therapeutic potential of herbal substances in cancer prevention and therapy is ongoing, with promising findings from laboratory and clinical research. Incorporating herbal medicines into integrative cancer care strategies may provide advantages over conventional therapy alone.

3. Holistic Healing and Empowerment: Dr. Sebi's holistic approach to healing extends beyond his specific nutritional and therapeutic suggestions to a broader philosophy of empowerment, selfcare, and overall wellbeing. Dr. Sebi enabled people to retake control of their health and follow therapeutic routes that align with their values and beliefs by encouraging them to take an active part in their health, make informed lifestyle choices, and create a deeper connection with nature.

Dr. Sebi's emphasis on the connectivity of mind, body, and spirit is consistent with the ideas of integrative medicine, which aims to treat the complete person rather than just the ailment. Dr. Sebi's teachings have helped bridge the gap between conventional and alternative approaches to treatment by emphasizing the significance of addressing physical, emotional, and spiritual aspects of health.

CONTINUING THE JOURNEY OF NATURAL HEALING

As we consider the future of natural healing, several significant themes emerge that will influence the progress of holistic medicine and its integration into mainstream healthcare.

1. Research and EvidenceBased Practice: Researching the safety, efficacy, and mechanisms of natural medicines is crucial for improving holistic medicine and obtaining acceptance in the medical community. Integrative treatments require rigorous scientific investigations, such as randomized controlled trials and metaanalyses, to develop evidencebased guidelines for clinical practice. Collaboration among academics, healthcare professionals, and complementary medicine practitioners is essential for developing and carrying out highquality studies that produce useful data and support evidencebased decisionmaking in patient care.

2. Education and Training: Incorporating holistic medicine education into medical school curricula, residency programs, and continuing medical education is crucial for educating healthcare providers to use integrative techniques in practice. By increasing healthcare professionals' understanding and respect for complementary therapies, we may increase patient access to safe, effective, evidencebased holistic care.

Interdisciplinary collaboration and communication among practitioners of conventional and complementary medicine, as well as ongoing professional development and peertopeer learning opportunities, are critical for promoting dialogue, sharing best practices, and advancing the field of integrated medicine.

3. PatientCentered Care: The idea of holistic medicine emphasizes empowering people to participate actively in their health and treatment decisions. By encouraging patients and healthcare providers to work together, we can improve patient engagement, satisfaction, and outcomes. Patientcentered care entails listening to patients' problems, values, and preferences; giving them correct information and tools to help them make educated decisions; and assisting them in executing tailored treatment plans that are aligned with their objectives and priorities.

4. Health Equity and Access: Providing equitable access to comprehensive healthcare services and resources is crucial for promoting health equity and reducing disparities in cancer treatment. To ensure that all people, regardless of socioeconomic status, race, ethnicity, or geographic location, have access to the full range of holistic healing modalities, efforts must be made to expand insurance coverage for integrative treatments, increase funding for complementary therapy research, and improve access to affordable, culturally competent care.

Communitybased initiatives, grassroots advocacy activities, and governmental reforms can all play important roles in improving health equity and fostering social justice in healthcare.

5. Global Collaboration and Knowledge Sharing: Collaboration among healthcare providers, researchers, policymakers, advocacy organizations, and community leaders is crucial for advancing natural healing and tackling global health challenges like cancer prevention and treatment. By sharing knowledge, resources, and best practices across borders and disciplines, we can tap into the global community's combined experience and skills to enhance health outcomes and promote overall wellbeing.

International forums, conferences, and networks are excellent venues for interdisciplinary collaboration, crosscultural exchange, and capacity building in holistic medicine. By encouraging global discourse, collaboration, and innovation, we can hasten the transition to a more holistic, patientcentered, and sustainable healthcare system.

Made in United States
Troutdale, OR
03/17/2025